HEALING PTSD

HEALING
PTSD

A CBT Workbook for Taking Back Your Life

Sabina Mauro, PsyD

ROCKRIDGE PRESS

Interior and Cover Designer: Rachel Haeseker
Photo Art Director/Art Manager: Tom Hood
Editor: Meera Pal
Production Editor: Ashley Polikoff

Illustration © 2020 Pavel Fuksa, p 6; Sergey Pekar/Shutterstock, cover and interior; Author photograph courtesy Violetta B Photography.

ISBN: Print 978-1-64739-835-4 | eBook 978-1-64739-532-2

R0

This book is dedicated to the survivors of trauma. Your strength inspires me every day. You are not alone.

Contents

Introduction

Life rarely goes as expected, but often we continue to thrive, doing the best that we can because we are equipped to deal with what life throws at us. But if you have been exposed to a life-threatening or traumatic event, life can become more challenging and you may find yourself "surviving" day to day rather than thriving.

The world can suddenly feel unsafe and dangerous. You may start to avoid situations that remind you of your trauma. Your days might become filled with thoughts about your trauma. Even your sleeping pattern may change because you have nightmares about the traumatic event. Life can feel out of your control.

If you have experienced any or all of these reactions, you may be struggling with posttraumatic stress disorder (PTSD). What this means is that right now PTSD may have control of your life. But you picked up this book because you are ready to learn how to regain control and live your best life. Imagine how empowered you will feel when you've completed this workbook and have the tools to successfully tackle painful memories.

These physical and psychological reactions can happen because your body and brain experienced more stress than they could handle at the time of the traumatic event and are unable to independently return to their previous level of functioning. But this does not have to be a permanent condition. The brain can be rewired. Even though the memory may remain, your response to the memory can be rewired.

The effects of your trauma might be dominating your life currently, making you feel as though you no longer have control. You might feel lost. You might feel that nobody can understand what you're going through. You might feel alone. There might be days when you feel defeated, when you can see no alternatives, when you feel that this struggle is meant to defeat you.

But you are not alone. The World Mental Health Survey of 70,000 people from 24 countries found that 70 percent of participants reported having experienced at least one traumatic event. Most likely, you have already come into contact with at least one other person who has experienced a traumatic event. However, you may not know that about them because trauma is not a part of daily conversation.

No matter where you currently find yourself in terms of coping with your trauma, there is always room for improvement. If you feel that you have been stuck on an endless path of struggle and suffering, take heart. There is a different path. A path of hope. A path that has been proven to help people reach their healthier, happier life. And this book will show you the way.

This book offers you proven and well-researched methods to help you learn how to move forward, as well as improve your well-being and quality of life. There is no right or wrong way to complete the exercises. There is no deadline for completion. Give yourself not one but multiple chances to go through this workbook. Connect with your thoughts, feel your emotions, and over time, past memories will become less scary.

Allow me to join you as your guide along the path toward a place known as posttraumatic growth. I am a psychologist, and for more than six years, I have treated trauma survivors exclusively. I have witnessed my clients make the transition from "surviving" to "thriving," or achieving posttraumatic growth. I have seen people heal. You, too, can heal.

I am going to accompany you on this PTSD journey by providing you with well-researched and proven therapy tools that I use with my clients so that you, too, can thrive. Throughout this book, I refer to you (or anyone who has experienced a trauma) as a trauma survivor because you survived the past and do not have to continue to "relive" it. You are a survivor.

Now let's conquer PTSD together.

How to Use This Book

This book is intended to help you manage the effects of a traumatic event in a healthy and productive manner. You will learn about PTSD, how it forms, and how you can live a happier life.

This book is not meant to self-diagnose or cure you of PTSD, but rather to offer you guidance based in cognitive behavioral therapy (CBT) and help you overcome painful and lingering effects of the traumatic experience. If you finish this workbook and still feel like you aren't at your optimal functioning, that is okay, because there are other resources available (see page 186).

This book will teach you about trauma and PTSD, introduce you to new concepts, and provide you with tools to overcome your PTSD. I recommend that in order to get the most benefit from this book, you work through each section before moving forward. Each section and exercise is designed to help you along the journey to getting your life back.

When you close this workbook, it does not mean that you are closing PTSD. Trauma recovery is a lifelong process, and there will likely be times when you feel that you have lost control of PTSD again. That is okay; you can always return to this workbook to regain that control.

My hope is that you will give yourself multiple chances to really reflect on your trauma and PTSD so you can heal and recover. The past (up until this moment) cannot be changed or undone. What can be changed is how you think, feel, and react to what happened to you. You have complete power and control to use the strategies in this workbook.

I hope that by the end of this book you will recognize that your trauma does not define who you are as a person and that the work you did in these pages has shaped you into a better, stronger, and more resilient survivor.

Please Note

This workbook will cause you to confront some painful and uncomfortable memories, but it should not cause feelings of self-harm or suicide. If at any point you have thoughts of suicide or self-harm, please call the National Suicide Prevention Lifeline at 1-800-273-8255.

You should also develop and follow a safety plan. Fill out this plan so you have it ready if you need it.

My Safety Plan

My warning signs include:

Thoughts: ....

....

Emotions: ....

....

Specific memories: ....

....

Body sensations: ....

....

Situations: ....

....

Behaviors: ....

....

Places I can go to feel safe: ....

....

1. ....

....

2. ....

....

3. ....

....

I can keep myself safe in my environment by making these things inaccessible to me:

1. ....
....

2. ....
....

3. ....
....

Things I can do to take my mind off my problems:

1. ....
....

2. ....
....

3. ....
....

I can reach out to the following person to talk about

My emotions: ....

My trauma: ....

My suicidal or self-harm thoughts: ....

This is one thing that is important and worth living for:

....

....

If I completed all these steps and still feel suicidal, I promise myself that I will pause this workbook, seek help, and return to this workbook when I am in a better mental place.

Part 1

Recognizing Trauma & PTSD

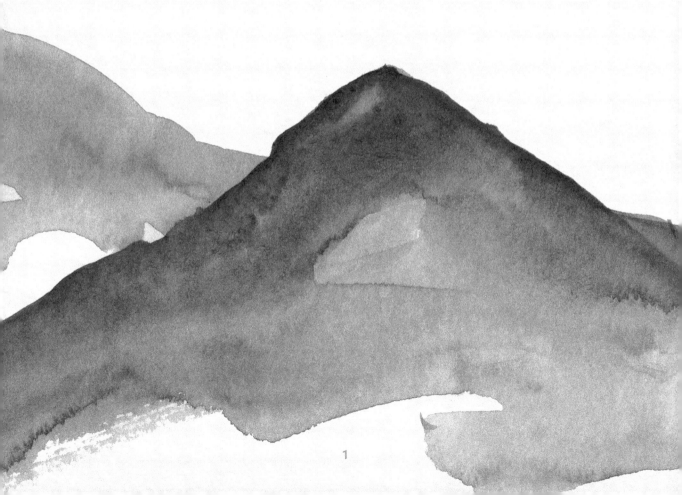

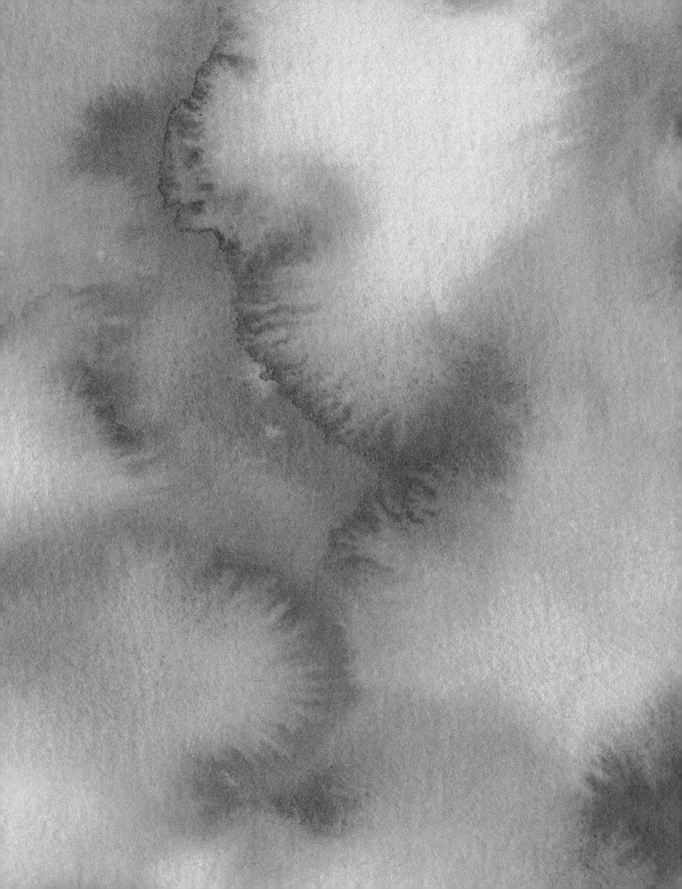

Chapter 1

Traumatic Events

In this chapter is an overview of trauma. The goal is to help you recognize that you are not alone. You will read about concepts that may or may not be new to you. By the end of this chapter, you will be able to:

- identify and describe trauma,

- recognize the different types of trauma,

- understand how trauma impacts the brain,

- learn how traumatic events impact your memory, and

- gain awareness of the types of strategy you use to manage your PTSD.

Ready? Let's go.

What Is Trauma?

The majority of us will at some point experience a traumatic event. In fact, trauma exposure is common throughout the world. In a 2017 study published in the *European Journal of Psychotraumatology*, a group of researchers conducted surveys in 24 countries and found that 70.4 percent of respondents experienced exposure to one or more traumas at some time.

Although exposure to a traumatic event may be common, only a small number of individuals develop posttraumatic stress disorder (PTSD), a mental health disorder that is given as a diagnosis to trauma survivors who have difficulty recovering after a traumatic event. PTSD is explained in more depth in chapter 2 (see page 13).

There are many factors apart from the traumatic event itself that predispose an individual to the development of PTSD. These factors are explained in chapter 2.

It's important to mention that some individuals do report experiencing a positive change after a traumatic event. This positive change is referred to as posttraumatic growth, which is discussed in chapter 12 (see page 159).

Trauma Defined

Psychological trauma is defined as one's response to an event that is perceived to be harmful or life-threatening and that causes negative physiological and/or psychological changes.

Trauma can be categorized as human-made (e.g., child abuse, domestic violence, and military-related trauma) or products of nature (e.g., earthquakes, tsunamis, and hurricanes). They can occur as one single traumatic event or as a series of multiple chronic events.

The effects of trauma can carry over from one generation to the next. This phenomenon has been referred to as *transgenerational trauma*. Examples include genocide and Holocaust survival.

Although there are numerous types of traumatic events that an individual or group of individuals can experience, the hallmark feature of traumatic events is that they are imprinted in our memory.

The Aftermath of Trauma

If you were asked to recall a specific emotional event from your past, you would have to make a conscious effort to play back the memory from your original vantage point. The area of the brain responsible for the recall of past events is known as *autobiographical memory*. You're able to recall these types of memories because, in general, emotional memories are encoded more vividly.

After highly emotional events, you may experience involuntary memories that come spontaneously and are usually unharmful. These memories are referred to as *intrusive memories* and are a common occurrence in day-to-day life. For example, a memory of your wedding day might "pop" into your head. This memory reminds you of how much you love your partner, and as a result of the memory, you experience happiness.

Intrusive memories can also be upsetting if they are recollections of traumatic events. Their frequency, vividness, or associated emotional distress make such memories the hallmark of psychological trauma. When intrusive thoughts and accompanying images of your past trauma randomly pop into your head, you'll often have a biological reaction that may include an increased heart rate, sweatiness, and difficulty concentrating. This intrusive memory may also elicit a physical reaction from you, such as you punching the wall or isolating yourself.

These types of intrusive memories are disruptive, cause increased physical and emotional arousal, and disconnect you from the present moment. A near-photographic memory of your traumatic event is referred to as a *flashbulb memory*. These intrusive images mirror your experience during the original event and can make you feel as though you've been transported back to the actual moment when the trauma occurred, thus making you feel like you are frequently "reliving" your trauma.

Your Brain & Trauma

Autobiographical memory and flashbulb memory are not the only parts of the brain that are hijacked after a traumatic event. Research has shown that trauma survivors show very specific changes in the brain. The brain of an individual who has been diagnosed with PTSD is more complex because different parts of the brain are activated during different traumatic events.

All trauma leaves its imprint on the brain. Research has shown that traumatic stress may disrupt the normal pattern of three specific areas of the brain: the amygdala, prefrontal cortex, and hippocampus. Once disrupted, these areas experience change and cannot communicate effectively. However, these changes are not permanent because the brain has the capacity to evolve and make new connections, a term referred to as *neuroplasticity*.   »

These are the main areas of the brain that experience change due to trauma:

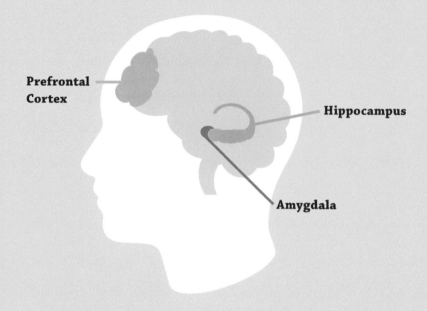

Amygdala: The amygdala is part of our "danger alertness." It's responsible for managing the emotional and behavioral responses needed for survival in the face of real or perceived threat. When the amygdala has identified something as threatening or dangerous, it becomes activated and biological changes occur: breathing quickens, heart rate increases, blood pressure goes up, pupils dilate, and appetite is suppressed. This is referred to as the "fight-or-flight" response, which is designed to protect us from threat or danger. During a traumatic event, the brain first activates the fight response, the ability for you to fight back. If this response is not an option, the brain automatically activates the flight response, the ability for you to run away or escape from the trauma. However, if neither the fight nor flight response is a viable option or if they become inactive due to the body being overwhelmed, the brain activates the "freeze" response, or the inability to fight or flee. It is at this point that the experience is considered trauma, because the response to threat did not work. Trauma survivors are more likely to have an overactive amygdala because of the powerful effect of a traumatic event; the emotional response that occurred during the traumatic event has been encoded by the amygdala.

Prefrontal cortex: The prefrontal cortex is located in the front of the brain and plays a significant role in reasoning, problem-solving, planning, memory, and aspects of emotional regulation. One of the responsibilities of the prefrontal cortex is to control the amygdala.

Because the prefrontal cortex is also disrupted after a traumatic event, it is unable to help the amygdala effectively process fear. Instead, the prefrontal cortex reacts by choosing the best course of action (frequently maladaptive behaviors) to get out of the misperceived danger.

Hippocampus: The hippocampus is primarily involved in memory and learning. It helps process information about your life experiences and stores it for later retrieval. The hippocampus also stores the memory of a traumatic event, which cannot be simply erased. When that memory is retrieved, it can feel as though the trauma is "real" and happening again. Research has shown that high levels of stress cause the hippocampus to shrink and become underdeveloped.

How I Cope with Trauma

Coping skills are strategies we use in response to a stressful situation, as part of an effort to adapt and maintain our psychological and physical well-being. The goal of this exercise is not to self-diagnose but to provide you with a baseline of your coping strategies as they relate to the traumatic event.

1. Are you coping more in healthy or unhealthy ways?

Although it's nearly impossible to turn to healthy coping skills 100 percent of the time, it's important to maintain healthier strategies for your well-being. At times you may even use an unhealthy coping strategy in conjunction with a healthy coping strategy. For example, you may frequently turn to your support system, but during a stressful situation, you may choose to isolate yourself for a few hours to cry. The important thing is being able to bounce back from an unhealthy coping strategy. Coping strategies are learned skills, and it is within your control to use them.

EXAMPLES OF HEALTHY COPING STRATEGIES	EXAMPLES OF UNHEALTHY COPING STRATEGIES
Healthy eating	Self-harm behavior
Talking about your problem	Drug or alcohol use
Using social support	Overeating/undereating
Contacting a mental health professional	Isolation
Problem-solving techniques	Sleeping too much/too little

2.   How do you cope with intrusive memories related to your
traumatic event?

We all experience intrusive memories. For some people, intrusive memories aren't bothersome. For trauma survivors, intrusive memories of the traumatic event can cause significant distress, especially because the memory occurs involuntarily.

If you are using healthy coping strategies the majority of the time to manage your intrusive thoughts, you would not rely on this workbook to help you heal. Trauma survivors fear intrusive memories and are scared to access them, which is why they turn to unhealthy coping strategies to temporarily escape the memories and unwanted feelings.

EXAMPLES OF HEALTHY COPING STRATEGIES	EXAMPLES OF UNHEALTHY COPING STRATEGIES
Talking about my memory	Avoiding talking about my memory
Not looking to distract myself from the memory	Intentionally suppressing the memory
Not being scared to access the memory	Being in denial about the memory
Labeling the memory as intrusive	Distracting myself to avoid experiencing the intrusive memory
Practicing mindfulness	
Experiencing the emotions	

3.   Do you use avoidant coping strategies?

Avoidant coping strategies involve intentionally avoiding stressors that may trigger a memory of your trauma, rather than confronting the stressors. Avoidance plays an important role in the development and maintenance of PTSD. These types of strategies limit how you process painful memories and the emotional reactions to those memories, thus preserving your PTSD.

EXAMPLES OF EMOTION-FOCUSED DISENGAGEMENT	EXAMPLES OF PROBLEM-FOCUSED DISENGAGEMENT
Being in denial about trauma	Emotional numbness
Avoiding anything related to the trauma	Self-criticism
Perceiving the trauma from my own perspective	Blaming myself for the trauma
	Rumination

4.   Are you actively coping with your trauma?

Active coping refers to dealing directly with your trauma and the ways in which the trauma has affected you. Active coping focuses on trying to control the pain and allows you to function despite the pain you are experiencing. *Passive coping* focuses on surrendering to pain over control.

At this present moment you are beginning to engage in active coping. By reading this book you are motivated to make changes and are reframing the meaning of your trauma. Keep going!

If you are using passive coping, it is okay; the coping skills you choose to use are within your control.

EXAMPLES OF ACTIVE COPING	EXAMPLES OF PASSIVE COPING
Seeing a mental health professional	Not confronting the trauma
Accepting the impact of trauma	Self-medicating
Reframing the meaning of your trauma	Not being motivated to make changes in your life

5. Which unhealthy coping strategies would you be willing to trade for healthy coping strategies?

List one unhealthy coping strategy you would be willing to trade for a healthy coping strategy. Try this one change as you work your way through the workbook.

UNHEALTHY COPING MECHANISMS I WANT TO TRADE . . .	. . . FOR THESE HEALTHY COPING MECHANISMS

Chapter 1 Takeaways

This chapter gave you an overview of trauma. To recap, here are the main points:

- It is well established that the majority of us at some point will experience a psychological traumatic event.

- Psychological trauma is the response to an event perceived to be harmful or life-threatening, causing physiological and psychological changes, as well as negative effects.

- Trauma can be a vicious cycle.

- Traumatic events cause intrusive (involuntary) memory recollection.

- Trauma causes changes in the brain.

This workbook will help you recognize that trauma is an obstacle that you can overcome. You will gain more insight and awareness into how your traumatic event has affected you and your well-being. You will also acquire tools to empower you to overcome your struggle with PTSD and regain control of your life.

It may have been hard for you to go through this chapter and recognize that you have been impacted by your trauma, but remember, you are in total control of your healing and recovery. The next chapter will introduce you to posttraumatic stress disorder (PTSD).

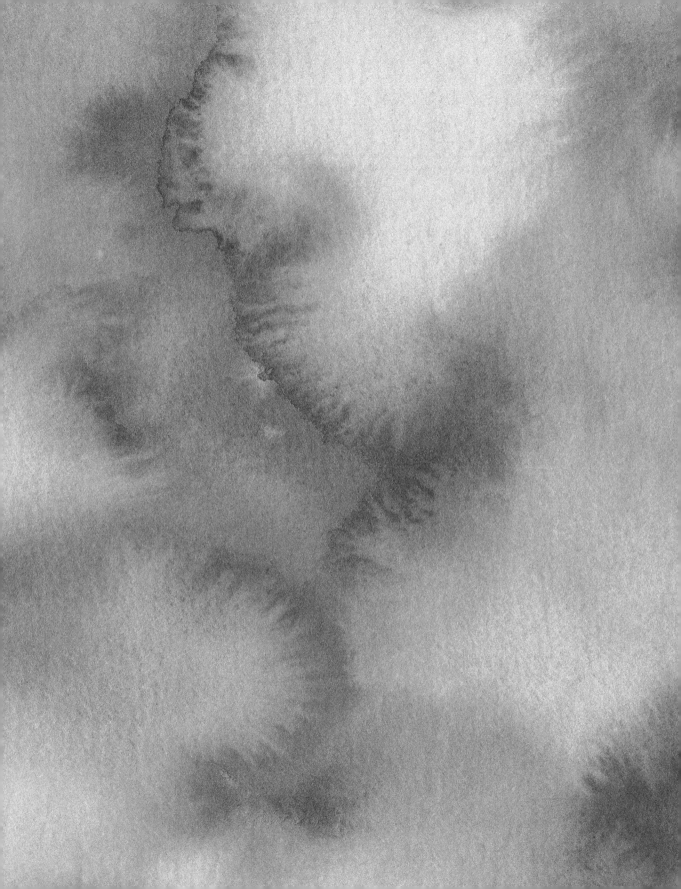

Chapter 2

Understanding PTSD

In chapter 1 you learned about trauma. In this chapter, you will learn how experiencing trauma can lead to the development of PTSD. I will introduce you to concepts with which you may not be familiar. The goal of this chapter is to familiarize you with PTSD and help you determine whether you may be struggling with it. By the end of this chapter, you will:

- know the history of PTSD,

- better understand PTSD,

- be able to identify symptoms of PTSD,

- know how common PTSD is, and

- determine if you may be struggling with PTSD.

   Ready? Let's go.

What Is PTSD?

Even though PTSD has been referred to as post-Vietnam syndrome, battle fatigue, and exhaustion, researchers are now aware that war veterans are not the only people who can experience trauma-like symptoms. In 1980, the American Psychiatric Association added PTSD to the third edition of its *Diagnostic and Statistical Manual of Mental Disorders (DSM-III)*. Since then, the diagnosis has been redefined over the years. In 2013, an important change occurred when PTSD was recategorized from an anxiety disorder to a trauma- and stressor-related disorder. As more research continues, it is possible that the diagnosis will again be revised.

As noted in chapter 1, even though a majority of people have experienced a traumatic event, less than 10 percent of the general population will develop PTSD. Trauma exposure alone is not the precursor to PTSD; certain factors prior to, during, and after the trauma play a part in the development of PTSD.

Factors prior to the trauma are referred to as *risk factors*. These include preexisting mental health conditions, a highly anxious personality trait (e.g., neuroticism), childhood trauma, previous exposures to trauma, lower levels of education, family history of substance abuse, or living in an urban setting. A 2013 study in the journal *Medical Care* found that racial and ethnic discrimination may play a part in the development of PTSD among African American and Latinx populations. Similar findings were published in 2019 in the journal *American Psychologist*. Another study published in 2014 found that Native Americans and Native Alaskans are also at greater risk for developing PTSD compared with their white counterparts.

Factors experienced during the trauma are referred to as *peritraumatic factors*. Some of these factors include the severity and nature of the trauma, the perceived life threat, and personal injury.

Although certain factors (e.g., adverse childhood experiences) place a trauma survivor at risk for PTSD, there are others that protect them from developing PTSD. These are referred to as *protective factors* and can be learned and developed. Examples include having a support network, seeking help, and healthy coping skills.

It is important to remember that PTSD may not present itself directly after a traumatic event. Some trauma survivors develop symptoms one month after the incident, for others this occurs a few months or even years after the traumatic event. Symptoms present themselves differently in each trauma survivor. For some, symptoms go away on their own. For others, symptoms continue to manifest and carry over into daily activities such as work, relationships, family, and school.

Remember, although PTSD may be currently present in your life, it does not have to run your life.

Do I Have PTSD?

PTSD is a disorder that is diagnosed by a mental health professional. Use this exercise as a guide to help you determine if you may be experiencing symptoms of PTSD. This exercise is not intended as a self-diagnosis tool, but to provide you with more awareness about possible symptoms.

1. In what ways does your brain continue to "remind" you about your traumatic event?

_____

_____

_____

_____

Because the memory of the traumatic event cannot simply be erased, it becomes imprinted on your brain. This memory is unwanted, unpleasant, and becomes intrusive. It can present itself through vivid images, nightmares, and distressing thoughts.

2. In what ways have you tried to "not remember" your trauma?

_____

_____

_____

_____

_____

The traumatic event is so powerful and painful that trauma survivors will seek alternative methods for "not remembering" the trauma. This can include avoiding people, places, sounds, odors, and other things that may trigger a memory.

3.   How has your view of yourself and the world changed since the traumatic event?

The negative impact of the trauma may cause the trauma survivor to develop a negative view of themselves in order to make sense of what just happened (e.g., I deserved it). They may also develop a distorted view of others (e.g., I can't trust other people) and a distorted worldview because trauma survivors may start to see the world as a dangerous and unsafe place.

4.   In what ways do you feel disconnected from emotions?

Trauma survivors may not be able to control their feelings. Emotional dysregulation can elicit aggressive behaviors and self-destructive behaviors. Remember, there is no right or wrong way to feel about your trauma. It is the processing of your emotions that is going to heal the wound successfully.

5. What are some everyday activities that have become challeng-
    ing? Why?

    _____

    _____

    _____

    _____

    _____

Trauma causes significant shock to your body. It can become difficult (or nearly impossible) to maintain a job or other responsibilities. You may have some good days, but most days you may feel like you cannot regain control of your life. Because your brain has been rewired to constantly be on the lookout for danger, everyday activities become challenging. Treating the PTSD will allow you to regain better functioning of your everyday activities.

6. How would you feel if you were diagnosed with PTSD?

    _____

    _____

    _____

    _____

    _____

Symptoms of PTSD are treatable. Your first step is to start with this book. If you feel that you are still unable to regain control of your PTSD, seek professional help.

Chapter 2 Takeaways

This chapter introduced you to PTSD, a diagnosis given after a traumatic event. To recap, here are the main points:

- Traumatic events alone do not place someone at risk for development of PTSD.

- War veterans are not the only trauma survivors reporting trauma-like symptoms.

- PTSD became an official diagnosis in 1980.

- Specific life challenges prior to a traumatic event are risk factors for developing PTSD.

- PTSD can occur at any point in life.

  In the next chapter, we will discuss the symptoms of PTSD in more depth.

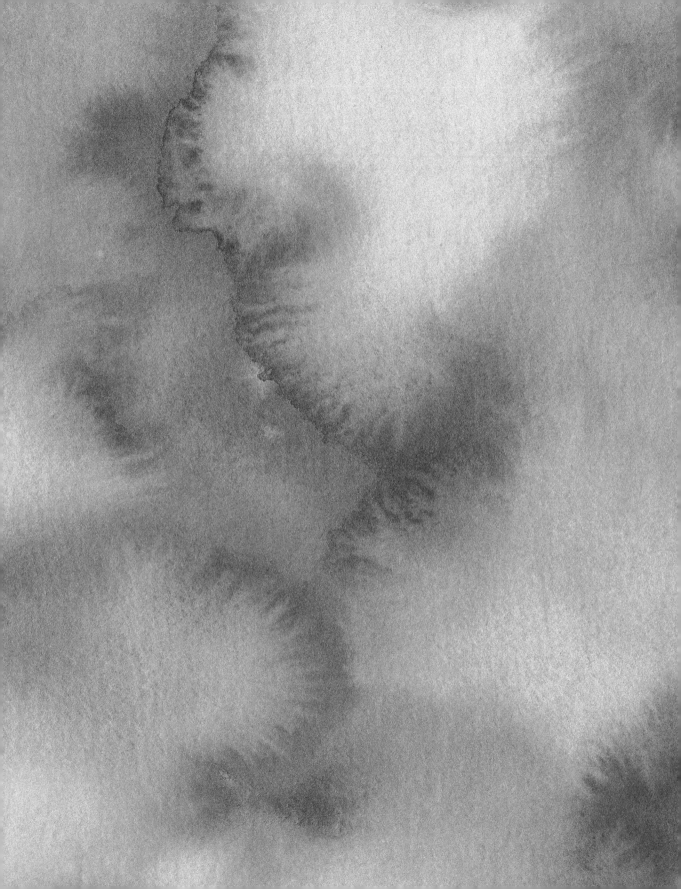

Chapter 3

Signs of PTSD

So far, you've learned about trauma and PTSD. We've covered describing a traumatic event, how PTSD evolved, and who is at risk for trauma exposure and PTSD. You should also have an idea of how you have reacted to your own trauma. In this chapter, we're going to:

- identify the symptoms of PTSD,

- get a better understanding of how PTSD is diagnosed,

- learn to identify triggers related to PTSD,

- develop an understanding of how PTSD has impacted you,

- learn that PTSD can co-occur with other mental health conditions, and

- understand the difference between PTSD and complex PTSD.

  Ready? Let's go.

Major PTSD Symptoms

Although a majority of individuals will experience a traumatic event in their lifetime, most are able to recover and return to their daily routines and lifestyle. However, for some, the symptoms persist and continue to impact areas of life, including work, relationships, family, and school.

As noted in chapter 2, PTSD was introduced as a diagnosis in 1980 by the American Psychiatric Association and was added to the third edition of the *Diagnostic and Statistical Manual of Mental Disorders* (*DSM-III*). The *DSM* is a handbook that is used by health care professionals in the United States to guide the diagnosis of mental health disorders.

In the latest edition, *DSM-5*, PTSD is categorized as a trauma- and stressor-related disorder. PTSD is diagnosed based on the following criteria:

- Exposure to a trauma

- Reexperiencing symptoms

- Avoidance

- Change in mood and thoughts

- Changes in arousal and reactivity

Children (over the age of six) and adults can be diagnosed with PTSD. In order to receive a diagnosis of PTSD, symptoms must be present for at least one month. However, it's important to note that although not every single symptom has to be present to meet the diagnosis, symptoms must cause impairment in other areas of life. If you do not meet the full criteria for PTSD but are experiencing trauma-like symptoms, you may be suffering from a different trauma- and stressor-related disorder.

The next section gives you a closer look at the *DSM-5* criteria for diagnosing PTSD. These symptoms are common reactions that are reported by trauma survivors, although each trauma survivor will experience symptoms differently. Becoming familiar with the specific descriptions of each criteria will help you better evaluate your own symptoms.

Exposure to Trauma

An essential first step to prescribe a diagnosis of PTSD is to determine if the individual has been exposed to trauma. Exposure to trauma is defined by the

DSM-5 as "actual or threatened death, serious injury, or sexual violence." According to the *DSM*, there are two types of qualifying exposures that an individual can experience: direct exposure or indirect exposure.

Direct exposure: This involves experiencing trauma firsthand and can also include witnessing a trauma as it occurs to someone else.

Indirect exposure: Learning that a traumatic event occurred to someone close to you is an example of indirect exposure. Being repeatedly exposed to or experiencing aversive details of a traumatic event is also a form of indirect exposure.

Indirect exposure to trauma can also be referred to as *vicarious trauma* or *secondary trauma* through a firsthand account or narrative of the event. Vicarious trauma can occur in professionals who work in high-stress and trauma-related fields, such as judges, rescue workers, police officers, doctors, mental health professionals, and abuse investigators. Familiar phrases used by these professionals include "burnout" and "compassion fatigue."

This type of trauma develops when workers in high-stress, trauma-related fields listen to painful memories or see disturbing images as they learn about a patient's traumatic experience. These images and memories then become a part of their own memory system.

Exposure to Trauma Checklist

DIRECT EXPOSURE	YES	NO
Have you experienced childhood maltreatment, such as neglect, sexual abuse, or physical abuse?		
Have you experienced intimate partner violence, such as physical, sexual, or emotional assault by a partner?		
Have you experienced someone dying in front of you?		
Have you experienced war-related trauma?		
Have you ever witnessed someone close to you experience abuse?		
Have you ever witnessed someone close to you experience a trauma?		
Have you directly experienced any other trauma? List: _____		

»

INDIRECT EXPOSURE	YES	NO
Have you learned that someone close to you experienced a trauma (e.g., a family member was diagnosed with cancer, best friend was shot and killed, partner was robbed at gunpoint)?		
Have you experienced any other indirect exposure? List: _____		

VICARIOUS/SECONDARY TRAUMATIZATION	YES	NO
Do you experience painful images and emotions associated with hearing about someone else's traumatic experiences?		
Do you experience painful images and emotions associated with your career responsibilities?		

If you answered no to all these questions, you do not meet the criteria for a PTSD diagnosis. A diagnosis of PTSD requires being exposed to a traumatic event. If you answered yes to at least one question, you meet the criteria for a potential PTSD diagnosis.

Intrusive Thoughts and Nightmares

Intrusive memories, flashbacks, and dissociation are all different aspects of reexperiencing symptoms. Spontaneous involuntary memories of past experiences are referred to as *intrusive memories*. As mentioned in chapter 1, intrusive memories are normal, occur after highly emotional events, and are usually unharmful. However, they may become distressing if they are of a traumatic nature. This reexperiencing is usually brief and is usually triggered by one of the five senses: vision, hearing, smell, taste, touch.

Some trauma survivors describe the memory of the trauma as "a movie replaying in my head." It can feel like the incident is taking place again and again in the present moment. This is referred to as *flashbacks*. An example of a flashback would include vivid details, and the trauma survivor may feel like they are drawn back into the traumatic experience.

Trauma survivors may also describe their trauma memory feeling so "real" that they lose touch with the present moment. This type of reexperiencing is referred to as *dissociation*. A trauma survivor who dissociates may experience feeling detached from the "here and now," exhibit identity confusion, or experience memory lapses such as forgetting important personal information.

Nightmares are also categorized as a reexperiencing symptom. Research suggests that nightmares are considered a trademark PTSD symptom, especially among both military combat veterans and trauma-exposed civilians. At least 70 percent of adults who have experienced a traumatic event develop nightmares. Nightmares based on traumatic events are emotionally intense, and trauma survivors are likely to wake up from them with strong and prolonged feelings of fear and anxiety. These individuals may cry in their sleep or wake up soaked in sweat. These trauma survivors are likely to employ behavior that will help them avoid falling asleep, such as staying up late or leaving the lights on.

Intrusive Thoughts and Nightmares Checklist

INTRUSIVE MEMORIES	YES	NO
Does your trauma randomly pop into your head?		
Do you fear this memory?		
Do you experience a physiological response (e.g., increased heart rate, sweatiness) when you have an intrusive thought?		
Does the intrusive memory cause distress?		
FLASHBACKS	YES	NO
Do you feel like you are reliving your trauma when you have a trauma memory?		
Does your intrusive memory include vivid and graphic details?		
Does your trauma memory feel like a movie replaying in your head?		
DISSOCIATION	YES	NO
Do you lose touch with reality when you think of your trauma?		
Do you "space out" when you have a trauma memory?		
Are you unable to remember anything for a period of time?		
Do you feel disconnected or detached from your emotions?		

»

NIGHTMARES	YES	NO
Do you have vivid dreams of your trauma?		
Do you wake up in a sweat or in fear?		
Do you avoid going to sleep because you do not want to have dreams of your trauma?		
Do you have dreams related to your trauma content?		
Do you have dreams of being hurt or killed?		

If you answered no to all these questions, you do not meet the criteria for intrusive thoughts or nightmare-related trauma symptoms. If you answered yes to at least one question, you meet the criteria for intrusive thoughts and nightmares.

Avoidance

Avoidance is a common symptom of PTSD and is used to prevent reminders of the trauma. Trauma survivors with this symptom will avoid anything related to their trauma-related thoughts, memories, triggers, and feelings. Avoidance is not a sign of weakness but a tool that trauma survivors have learned to use in order to escape their trauma-related symptoms. However, these avoidance-like behaviors become unhelpful when they begin to interfere with other areas of life.

Emotions are real. When we experience an unpleasant event, we want to avoid anything that reminds us of that event. "I don't want to think about it" is a common avoidant strategy to suppress the emotional response of an upsetting event. However, it's important to remember that emotions provide critical information about your surroundings, which improves your chances for survival. For example, fear allows you to assess danger and threats, sadness usually elicits help from others, and anxiety warns you that something unexpected may happen.

Ongoing avoidance is likely to have negative consequences for your well-being. By avoiding your feelings, you are not effectively coping with the underlying problem. Avoiding uncomfortable emotions requires a lot of energy on a daily basis and typically leads to the emotions becoming stronger over time.

Although your trauma is real, the memory of it is just that—a memory. Even though you may have deliberately tried to suppress the trauma, your body and brain continue to remind you that it happened. Trauma survivors will look for ways to avoid these traumatic memories. In order to avoid potential cues or triggers, survivors will likely withdraw from people, places, situations, conversations, activities, and objects. They will often say things like, "My trauma doesn't bother me," "There's no point thinking about it," or "I've moved on."

Avoidance Checklist

AVOIDANCE OF EMOTIONS	YES	NO
Do you avoid trauma-related feelings?		
Do you find other ways to cope with your trauma-related feelings?		
Have you ever expressed feeling "numb"?		
AVOIDANCE OF MEMORIES	YES	NO
Do you avoid trauma-related memories?		
Do you find other ways to cope with trauma-related memories?		
Do you find yourself frequently stating, "I can't remember what happened"?		
AVOIDANCE OF THOUGHTS	YES	NO
Do you avoid trauma-related thoughts?		
Do you find yourself frequently stating, "I don't think about it"?		
TRIGGERS	YES	NO
Do you avoid people who remind you of your trauma?		
Do you avoid conversations that remind you of your trauma?		
Do you avoid relationships because of your trauma?		
Do you avoid places that remind you of your trauma?		
Do you avoid any objects (e.g., foods, scented products, clothing) that remind you of the trauma?		

If you answered no to all these questions, you do not meet the criteria for avoidance symptoms. If you answered yes to at least one question, you meet the criteria for avoidance symptoms.

Changes in Mood and Thoughts

Trauma survivors may develop a negative thinking pattern as a result of a traumatic event. Often, these negative thoughts play a role in keeping the PTSD going. Research suggests that trauma survivors are likely to develop a negative view of themselves and the world. For example, trauma survivors may view themselves as less worthy and develop a view that bad things happen to good people and that the world is unsafe.

It is not uncommon for trauma survivors to blame themselves for the trauma they experienced. Due to recurring intrusive thoughts and memories, they are forced to relive the event and think about what they could have done or said differently. Often, trauma survivors attempt to find meaning in the trauma. They do so by blaming themselves and believe they brought the trauma upon themselves. Trauma survivors may develop persistent negative emotional states such as fear, anger, shame, guilt, and self-focused disgust.

Following a traumatic event, survivors may experience a sudden or gradual loss of interest in pleasurable activities. Their intrusive memories and triggers may become so overwhelming that they lose motivation to do things that once brought them joy.

These feelings can also cause trauma survivors to separate themselves from family and friends. They often feel different from others and believe that others will not understand their experiences. Often, survivors of childhood abuse or domestic violence have experienced a significant sense of betrayal and feel they cannot rely on or trust anyone, leading to even more isolation.

Sometimes, trauma survivors experience difficulty in accepting positive emotions. This may be because emotions lead to physical sensations. Because survivors already have increased physical sensations, they can't distinguish between the sensations that occur during positive and negative emotions.

Changes in Mood and Thoughts Checklist

NEGATIVE SELF-VIEW	YES	NO
Do you view yourself in a negative way?		
Is it hard to find positive qualities about yourself?		
Do you view yourself as worthless or less deserving?		
Do you view the world as unsafe?		
Do you criticize yourself?		
Do you have more negative than positive views of yourself?		
Do you have more negative than positive views of the world?		
SELF-BLAME	**YES**	**NO**
Do you blame yourself for your trauma?		
NEGATIVE EFFECT	**YES**	**NO**
Do you feel ashamed because of your trauma?		
Do you feel embarrassed because of your trauma?		
Are you frequently in fear?		
Do you feel angry most of the time?		
Is it hard to experience positive feelings?		
DIMINISHED INTEREST IN ACTIVITIES	**YES**	**NO**
Since your trauma, have you lost interest in things?		
Since your trauma, is it hard to find pleasure in anything?		
POOR RELATIONSHIPS	**YES**	**NO**
Since your trauma, is it hard to trust others?		
Since your trauma, do you feel "different" from others?		
Since your trauma, do you feel that nobody can understand you?		
Since your trauma, do you feel like there is no one you can rely on?		

»

INABILITY TO EXPERIENCE POSITIVE EMOTIONS	YES	NO
Is it hard to experience positive feelings?		
Do you experience more negative versus positive feelings?		
Is it hard to experience joy or happiness?		

If you answered no to all these questions, you do not meet the criteria for changes in mood and thoughts. If you answered yes to at least one question, you meet the criteria for changes in mood and thoughts.

Anger, Arousal, and Reactivity

Arousal symptoms are some of the most common symptoms experienced by trauma survivors. They can include things like irritability and aggression, which are valid emotional experiences until several things change:

- Emotional regulation

- Frequency

- Duration

- Severity

Often, these types of emotional difficulties arise with little to no provocation. Unhealed wounds can trigger wide swings in mood and emotions. These wide shifts begin to take over and show up in different settings, such as work, relationships, family, or public places. They also go from showing up every once in a while to showing up more often than not.

Research has shown that in the absence of helpful coping tools, PTSD can result in risky or unhealthy behaviors. Examples of these types of behaviors include deliberate self-harm, suicidal attempts, substance abuse, and practicing unsafe sex.

No matter what the situation is, trauma survivors are always in hypervigilance mode, constantly scanning their surroundings. They often feel like nothing is safe unless they can assess it themselves. They are frequently looking for cues that their trauma is about to recur. These cues could include clothing, odors, or noises. If any of those cues are present, their body enters survival mode, activating the fight-or-flight response.

Because trauma survivors already have a heightened fear response, they are also likely to have a heightened startle response. Trauma survivors may become easily startled or easily jumpy when a trauma cue has been identified. For example, a simple loud noise may trigger a combat veteran with PTSD to become easily startled.

Trauma survivors are likely to experience poor concentration as the traumatic event continuously hijacks their brain. Because the individual is unable to be present in the moment, poor concentration starts to impact other areas of life, including being able to focus on and hold a conversation.

One of the more common effects of experiencing a traumatic event is difficulty sleeping. An estimated 80 to 90 percent of trauma survivors complain of having sleep-related problems. Trouble with sleeping usually occurs when the individual intentionally avoids sleep so that they don't experience nightmares.

Anger, Arousal, and Reactivity Checklist

IRRITABILITY AND AGGRESSION	YES	NO
Do you feel angry all the time?		
Do you use phrases such as "lash out," "short temper," or "blackout"?		
Do you feel irritable all the time?		
MALADAPTIVE BEHAVIOR	YES	NO
Have you ever intentionally cut yourself to escape your trauma?		
Have you intentionally scratched/hit yourself to escape your trauma?		
Have you used drugs or alcohol to avoid your trauma?		
Have you been hypersexual (e.g. sex with multiple partners, unprotected sex)?		
Have you restricted your food intake, binged, or purged?		
HYPERVIGILANCE	YES	NO
Do you frequently pay attention to your surroundings?		
Do you frequently feel "on edge"?		
Do you feel unsafe at all times?		
Is it hard to trust others?		

»

HEIGHTENED STARTLE RESPONSE	YES	NO
Do you become easily startled?		
Do you become easily jumpy?		
DIFFICULTY CONCENTRATING	YES	NO
Is it hard to focus because of your trauma?		
Do your intrusive memories prevent you from staying focused?		
Is it hard to maintain a conversation because you are thinking about your trauma?		
Is it hard to perform simple tasks without losing focus because you are thinking of your trauma?		
DIFFICULTY WITH SLEEP	YES	NO
Have you ever tried to avoid sleep because of nightmares?		
Do you fear going to sleep because of your trauma?		

If you answered no to all these questions, you do not meet the criteria for arousal symptoms. To meet the criteria, you must experience at least two symptom clusters (e.g., hypervigilance and maladaptive behavior).

Anxiety, Depression, and Panic Attacks

It is well documented that PTSD can occur simultaneously with other mental health disorders, the most common being anxiety, depression, and panic disorder. About 80 percent of individuals with PTSD have a co-occurring mental health diagnosis. PTSD can lead to disorders that share similar symptoms but have their own causes, characteristics, and symptoms.

Anxiety: It's possible that trauma survivors may develop symptoms of anxiety, because some symptoms overlap. Both PTSD and anxiety disorders have physiological reactions, avoidance behaviors, distorted thinking, sleep disturbance, excessive worry and apprehension, and arousal reactions. It is important to share with your mental health professional that you have a trauma history so that your symptoms are not misinterpreted as anxiety symptoms.

Depression: Roughly 50 percent of individuals diagnosed with PTSD also suffer from major depression. In fact, there are many trauma symptoms that may be misdiagnosed as depression because many of the symptoms overlap. These symptoms include diminished interest, distorted thoughts, guilt, sleep disturbance, memory impairment, and trouble concentrating. Because trauma symptoms can overlap with depression, it is important that your mental health professional be aware of your trauma so that the appropriate symptoms are treated.

Panic attacks: Panic attacks and PTSD have shared symptoms, including chronic hyperarousal, hypervigilance, and somatic reactivity. Many trauma survivors report experiencing a panic attack during the traumatic event itself. A 2012 study published in the *European Journal of Psychotraumatology* found that panic attacks in trauma survivors are triggered by the fear of trauma memories, the fear of being harmed again, and the inability to control the trauma memories.

Panic attacks after a traumatic event usually occur due to an internal or external cue that later becomes a trigger for the attacks. In other words, a trauma survivor associates reminders of the threat (e.g., the smell of an orange) with fear (the learned response). In this example, each time the trauma survivor comes in contact with anything related to an orange, the trauma survivor becomes fearful and experiences a panic attack.

It is important that your mental health professional is aware of your trauma history so that treatment is targeted toward the trauma and not just panic disorder. Research has found that those with a panic disorder interpret their panic attacks differently than those with a history of trauma. Someone who experienced a traumatic event and has been diagnosed with PTSD fears the consequences of trauma memories.

Do I Have More Than PTSD?

Use this exercise as a guide to determine if you are struggling with a mental health disorder in addition to PTSD. Again, the goal of this exercise is not to self-diagnose but instead to reflect on your symptoms.

ANXIETY	YES	NO
Do you worry excessively?		
Do you feel restless?		
Do you have sleep problems?		
Do you have muscle tension?		
Do you have fatigue?		
DEPRESSION	YES	NO
Do you suffer from feelings of worthlessness or hopelessness?		
Have you had sleep changes?		
Have you had appetite changes?		
Have you had suicidal thoughts?		
Have you lost interest in activities you once enjoyed?		
Have you had feelings of guilt?		
Do you feel more tired than usual?		
PANIC ATTACKS	YES	NO
Do you have "attacks" of intense fear or discomfort for no apparent reason?		
If you answered yes, do you experience sensations such as sweatiness, a pounding heart, trembling, shaking, nausea, or chest pain?		
Do you fear losing control?		

If you answered yes to most of these questions, you may potentially be struggling with a mental health disorder in addition to PTSD. Please remember that only a mental health professional can diagnose you with these mental health conditions. Remember, whether you are struggling with PTSD or a combination of PTSD and other mental health disorders, they are treatable!

If you seek professional help, make sure to let your mental health provider know that you have a trauma history so that appropriate symptoms are addressed. People generally experience improved symptoms when the conditions are treated together.

Substance Abuse

Research has found that nearly half of all people diagnosed with PTSD also suffer from a substance abuse disorder. Trauma survivors may use drugs or alcohol as a way to escape from or cope with their traumatic event. However, because traumatic memories and feelings cannot be erased, the more they surface, the more likely it is that the trauma survivor will turn to drugs and/or alcohol to self-medicate.

According to the self-medication hypothesis, traumatic memories are distressing, so in order to avoid or escape the distress, trauma survivors rely on drugs or alcohol. By self-medicating, trauma survivors feel that their symptoms are "manageable." They feel in control of their symptoms by altering their response to their trauma through drugs and alcohol. Initially, self-medication may provide a sense of calm or relaxation when trauma triggers or memories arise, but in the long run it can lead to even greater problems.

Substance Abuse Checklist

Use this checklist to help you determine if your drug or alcohol use is problematic.

SUBSTANCE ABUSE	YES	NO
Do you have cravings to use drugs or alcohol?		
Do you want to cut down or stop but have difficulty doing so?		
Do you take drugs/alcohol in increasingly larger amounts or for longer periods of time?		
Has the use of drugs/alcohol impaired other areas of your life?		
Do you continue to use drugs/alcohol even if it causes problems in your relationships?		
Do you use drugs/alcohol even when it puts you in danger?		
Do you continue to use drugs/alcohol even if you have a physical or psychological condition?		
Do you experience withdrawal symptoms when you don't use drugs/alcohol?		

If you answered yes to most of the questions, you may be struggling with a substance abuse disorder. Just like mental health disorders, substance abuse disorders can be treated. If you are self-medicating to treat your PTSD, there are healthier, better, and adaptive coping skills. Please reach out to a substance abuse professional.

Take Back Your Life

PTSD affects everyone differently. Not all individuals will experience and process PTSD in the same manner. Although PTSD impacts your psychological well-being, it can also impact other areas of your life, including relationships, work, academics, and parenting. In the space provided, describe how PTSD has impacted your life.

Relationships (spouse, partner, friendships, family, etc.):

....

....

....

....

Work (if applicable):

....

....

....

....

School/Academics (if applicable):

....

....

....

....

Parenting (if applicable):

....

....

....

....

Other areas of your life:

....

....

....

....

Look back at what you wrote and notice how PTSD has controlled these areas of your life. Now imagine that you are able to fast-forward to successfully completing this workbook, conquering PTSD, and being in control of your life. Describe what you would see if you were able to fast-forward your life.

Relationships (spouse, partner, friendships, family, etc.):

....

....

....

....

Work (if applicable):

....

....

....

....

School/Academics (if applicable):

....

....

....

....

Parenting (if applicable):

....

....

....

....

Other areas of your life:

....

....

....

....

Getting Professional Help

After a traumatic event, it's not uncommon for someone's life to be momentarily disrupted. Eventually, many are able to regain control of daily functions. However, some trauma survivors do go on to develop PTSD and have greater difficulty managing their symptoms on their own. Their trauma may begin to dominate not just their thoughts and actions, but all areas of their life.

Healing and recovery from trauma is possible and you, too, can overcome your struggle. One of the hardest steps in beginning on your road to recovery will be reaching out to a professional, but once you're on that road, the journey becomes beautiful.

Here are some resources you can refer to for additional help:

WEBSITE	OFFERS
adaa.org (Anxiety and Depression Association of America)	Information and resources related to anxiety and depression.
apa.org (American Psychological Association)	Information related to the field of psychology.
griefnet.org (GriefNet)	Resources and information related to grief and access to over 50 online grief support groups for both children and adults.
mhanational.org (Mental Health America) mhanational.org/self-help-tools	Information and resources on mental health. The second link includes access to self-help tools such as screening tools and worksheets.
nami.org/home (National Alliance on Mental Illness)	Information related to mental health, including resources for the LGBTQ population.
ncadv.org (National Coalition Against Domestic Violence)	Resources for survivors of domestic violence.
nctsn.org (The National Child Traumatic Stress Network)	Information and resources related to childhood trauma.
nimh.nih.gov (National Institute of Mental Health)	Research on mental health and information about mental health disorders.
ptsd.va.gov (US Department of Veterans Affairs, National Center for PTSD)	Information and resources for veterans with PTSD.
samhsa.gov (Substance Abuse and Mental Health Services Administration)	Information related to substance abuse and mental health.
suicidepreventionlifeline.org (National Suicide Prevention Lifeline)	Phone numbers for free and confidential emotional support.

PTSD vs. Complex PTSD

In order to understand the difference between PTSD and Complex PTSD, we must first understand the difference between acute trauma and complex trauma.

Acute trauma: This involves exposure to a single event, such as a car crash.

Complex trauma: This involves exposure to repeated and prolonged trauma, such as living in a war zone, genocide, torture, or any form of abuse. This type of trauma is more pervasive, invasive, and occurs for a prolonged time. Individuals with complex trauma are likely to display greater complications than individuals exposed to acute trauma.

Complex PTSD

Complex PTSD, or C-PTSD, is considered a sibling of PTSD because both occur after a traumatic event. On the surface, both have similar symptoms. However, the debilitating effects of C-PTSD can be more enduring and extreme than PTSD.

The main difference between the two types of PTSD is the duration of the trauma. Additionally, PTSD can be described as a fear-based disorder whereas C-PTSD is described as involving chronic and repeated traumas. It is well documented that a history of childhood abuse can cause an individual to develop C-PTSD.

C-PTSD in children and adolescents can also be described as a developmental trauma disorder because the traumatic events occur in the context of a developing brain. During infancy, it is important for a baby to form healthy bonds with their primary caregiver, as a means of safety, security, and trust. A healthy bond between a baby and a caregiver (also referred to as a secure attachment) allows the developing brain to form trusting relationships, appropriate emotional regulation, and stability. Disruptions during the process of forming these healthy bonds can result in the brain rewiring and reprogramming how the child sees themselves and their relationships with others.

Symptoms of C-PTSD

In addition to the symptoms of PTSD (reexperiencing trauma, arousal, and reactivity; changes in mood and thoughts; and avoidance), C-PTSD symptoms also include challenges with:

- **Emotions:** Difficulty expressing, controlling, and recognizing emotions. Someone with C-PTSD may display persistent sadness, explosive anger, or emotional "numbness."
- **Self-perception:** A negative view of self, frequent self-blame, and frequent feelings of guilt.

- **Relationships:** Isolation, abrupt endings to relationships, ongoing unhealthy relationships, difficulty trusting others, and discomfort with intimacy.
- **Memories:** Includes dissociation, inability to recall memories, and feelings of reliving the trauma.
- **Biological reactions:** In addition to the common somatic symptoms (e.g., increased heart rate), over time, trauma survivors report tension headaches, gastrointestinal disturbances, fibromyalgia, and abdominal, back, or pelvic pain.
- **Beliefs:** Changes in beliefs about self, others, and the world.

Although C-PTSD is not recognized as a diagnosis in the *DSM-5*, it is recognized by the World Health Organization (WHO). In 2018, WHO recognized C-PTSD as a separate condition from PTSD and included the diagnosis in the *International Statistical Classification of Diseases and Relational Health Problems (ICD-11)*, a globally used diagnostic tool. Although C-PTSD is recognized globally, it is not the prominent focus of this workbook. If you would like more information on C-PTSD, you can find it at CPTSDFoundation.org.

Chapter 3 Takeaways

. . . .

This chapter provided you with a closer look at the specific symptoms of PTSD. To recap, here are the main points:

- In the United States, PTSD is recognized as a trauma- and stressor-related disorder.

- To meet the criteria for PTSD, symptoms must be present for a minimum of one month and you must have been exposed to a traumatic event, directly or indirectly.

- PTSD symptoms are based on four general clusters: avoidance, reexperiencing, arousal and reactivity, and changes in mood and thoughts. Symptoms must also impair other domains of life (e.g., work, relationships).

- It's common for individuals with PTSD to experience co-occurring mental health conditions, including depression, anxiety, and substance abuse.

- PTSD and other mental health disorders are treatable.

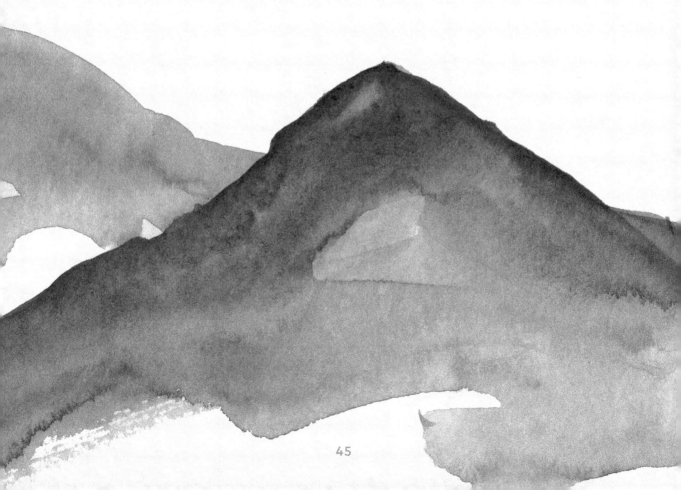

Part 2

Bring CBT into Your Life

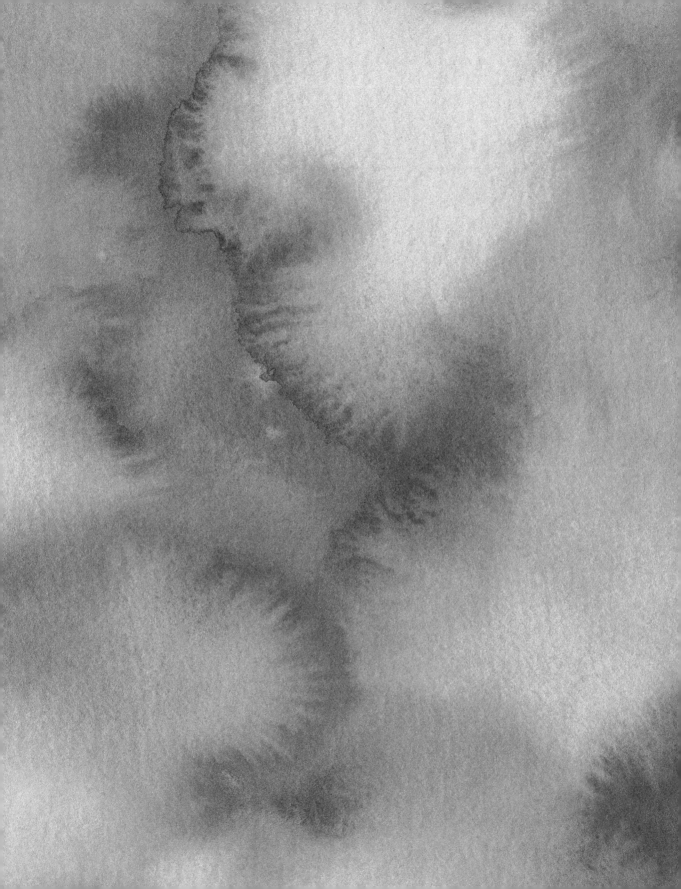

Chapter 4

Cognitive Behavioral Therapy

Mental health professionals use a variety of techniques to help individuals reduce their symptoms and improve their quality of life. There is a wide range of approaches available in the treatment of mental health diagnoses, including PTSD. Cognitive behavioral therapy (CBT) has been proven to be an effective treatment. In this chapter, you will:

- gain an understanding of how CBT is implemented,

- understand how CBT is effective for PTSD,

- learn about the benefits of CBT,

- increase your knowledge about other effective treatments for PTSD,

- define evidence-based treatment, and

- become aware of how PTSD has impacted your life.

   Ready? Let's go.

Why CBT for PTSD?

CBT has been shown to be effective in targeting PTSD symptoms arising from various different traumatic experiences, including adult survivors of terrorism, war trauma, sexual assault, traffic accidents, refugee status, and disasters. This treatment has also been effective in treating childhood and adolescent traumas. In fact, CBT has been recommended by the American Psychological Association, the leading scientific and professional organization representing psychology, as the "gold standard" of treatment modality for adults diagnosed with PTSD.

What Is CBT?

Developed by Albert Ellis and Aaron T. Beck, CBT is a style of "talk therapy" that is short term, structured, and problem focused. The therapist and trauma survivor work together in a collaborative problem-solving process. In its simplest form, CBT aims to teach patients to be their own therapists by helping them recognize and change unhelpful thought patterns that have a negative influence on emotions and behaviors.

CBT is based on the cognitive model, which emphasizes that it's not the situation or life event (i.e., the traumatic event) itself that affects us, but the meaning that we give to the situation or life event. In other words, the way we think of the situation influences and leads to certain emotional reactions and behaviors. The psychological impact of the traumatic event stems from trauma-related thinking patterns that then influence trauma-related emotional reactions and behaviors.

How Does CBT Help?

According to the emotional processing theory, fear is an emotional response represented in memory as a "network" to avoid or escape danger. This "fear network" consists of three structures to help someone assess their safety:

1. **Fear stimulus:** Anything that poses a fear to the individual (e.g., heights)

2. **Fear response:** The physiological response (e.g., increased heart rate)

3. **Meaning associated with stimulus and response:** Pairing the fear stimulus with fear response (e.g., heights are dangerous, and a fast heartbeat means I am afraid)

Here is an example of how this emotional processing theory is applied to a 20-year-old sexual assault trauma survivor:

1. **Fear stimulus:** An adult male

2. **Fear response:** An increased heart rate

3. **Meaning:** Because I have an increased heart rate, adult men are dangerous.

When a fear is realistic, we react with appropriate responses. Individuals with PTSD develop an unhealthy and unhelpful "fear network" because they develop unrelated associations between the three components. This is when trauma reminders, which are typically harmless, become threatening and cause physiological symptoms. Then the trauma survivor perceives the world to be dangerous. CBT addresses the unhelpful, unhealthy fear response by changing the associations.

In trauma work, repetitive exposure to trauma memories and trauma-related fears in a safe environment (such as therapy) can help reduce a survivor's PTSD and help them confront their fears. Successful treatment must first activate the "fear network" so that new learning may occur (e.g., not all adult males are dangerous) and replace old, unrealistic learning.

Studies have identified trauma-related thoughts about the self and the world as a core feature of PTSD. After a trauma survivor is exposed to trauma, they often develop post-trauma beliefs that influence how they think about themselves (e.g., I deserve this), about others (e.g., I cannot trust anyone), and about the world (e.g., the world is a dangerous place). These negative trauma-related thoughts "pop" into their head in response to a trigger and are referred to as *automatic thoughts*. Automatic thoughts have interchangeably been referred to as *thinking errors*, *maladaptive thoughts*, or *irrational thoughts*.

Automatic thoughts contribute to an ongoing perception of threats and have been shown to be associated with PTSD. CBT attempts to identify, challenge, and replace these maladaptive thoughts with more objective and realistic thoughts.

Although a range of emotions is present during and after trauma, survivors commonly experience five emotional responses: fear, anger, guilt, shame, and sadness. Fear arises during the immediate threat of trauma, whereas anger, guilt, shame, and sadness are frequently reported following the traumatic event.

In order to function, survivors usually try to make sense of the traumatic event by organizing their experience in a coherent way. This usually means engaging in unhelpful or unhealthy strategies to avoid negative thoughts and memories.

CBT can help someone with PTSD specifically address their avoidance and escapist behaviors, and help reestablish alternative, healthier behaviors.

The Benefits of CBT

CBT can be a powerful tool to help you win your battle with PTSD. It is a short-term treatment, which suggests that your PTSD symptoms will be addressed fairly quickly, and your quality of life can improve within a short amount of time. Additionally, studies have shown that CBT can help reduce PTSD symptoms for up to 12 months.

CBT allows trauma survivors to develop a sense of control over their thoughts, feelings, and behaviors. It teaches you how to be your own therapist in order to conquer your symptoms.

How PTSD Affects My Life

This exercise will help you gain better awareness of how PTSD has affected your life. This is not a self-diagnosis of PTSD, but is instead an exercise to help you recognize how PTSD has taken control of your life by reflecting on how your thoughts, emotions, and behaviors influence each other.

1.   Describe how your thoughts have changed since developing PTSD.

_____

_____

_____

_____

_____

We all have beliefs about self, others, and the world. These beliefs are influenced by our environment and experiences. After a traumatic event, you may experience shattered beliefs about yourself (e.g., I am incompetent, worthless) and the world (e.g., it is unsafe, dangerous). Eventually these negative distortions become part of your daily thoughts. However, these beliefs are not permanent, and with the right tools and strategies, maladaptive beliefs can be changed to adaptive thinking patterns.

2.   Describe how your emotions have changed since developing PTSD.

_____

_____

_____

_____

_____

Although it is not uncommon to develop a strong emotional reaction to a horrible event, trauma survivors are likely to have negative emotional states. As research has demonstrated, common trauma emotions include fear, anger, guilt, shame, and sadness. Each of these emotions can be experienced in multiple ways, and each emotion can be triggered by various things.

3.   Describe how your behaviors have changed since developing PTSD.

_____

_____

_____

_____

_____

Trauma survivors will evaluate their automatic thoughts, and emotional reactions will influence behavioral reaction. Trauma survivors are likely to engage in risky behavior (e.g., substance use, self-harm, physical aggression) that prevents them from changing negative appraisals and trauma memories.

4.   In what ways do you try to manage your PTSD?

_____

_____

_____

_____

_____

Some trauma survivors feel like they have lost control of their life. As such, they feel that they can control their PTSD by finding unhealthy ways to escape from their painful memories and unpleasant emotions.

5.   On a scale from 0 (low) to 10 (high), how would you rate your trauma-related fear?

0   1   2   3   4   5   6   7   8   9   10

Trauma survivors are likely to develop an unhealthy "fear network." They often have difficulty distinguishing trauma-related threats from actual threats and develop a heightened level of fear response. Exposure to feared situations in a safe environment can help survivors identify and change the distorted fear.

6.   How would your life be different if you did not have PTSD?

PTSD may have impacted your life, but you can take back control. You have the power to make that change. You cannot change the chapters that have already been written, but you are in total control of the next chapter of your life. In fact, you just wrote the next chapter of your life.

What Does Evidence-Based Treatment Mean?

Cognitive behavioral therapy is a type of evidence-based practice (EBP), which means that research has proven it to be a type of therapy that works. CBT treatments have been studied through the scientific process, submitted to the scientific community, and results have been replicated. This next section will review specific EBPs for treatment in PTSD. CBT is used as an umbrella term for a number of different treatments. CBT treatments for PTSD can be divided into trauma-focused and non-trauma-focused treatments:

Trauma-focused treatments concentrate on direct and detailed memory of the trauma and/or the meaning of the memory. Treatments that specifically target the memory of the trauma are referred to as *exposure therapy*. Exposure therapy is recommended as the first-line treatment because these specific treatments have been well researched and are proven effective.

Non-trauma-focused treatments target PTSD without focusing on trauma, thoughts, or feelings. Non-trauma-focused treatments offer strategies aimed at anxiety management and/or problem-solving. Trauma-focused treatments lead to stronger results than non-trauma interventions, although both are effective.

Not every trauma survivor needs trauma-focused treatment. For some, a combination of different CBT techniques may reduce their symptoms, whereas others may see benefits from a specific type of treatment. The descriptions provided are not meant for you to determine the best treatment for yourself, but are meant to provide you with information about each treatment. Only your therapist can determine the best treatment for you based on your unique combination of factors, such as severity of symptoms and past treatment experience, for example.

Trauma-Focused Treatments

Prolonged Exposure (PE) Therapy is the most well-researched and well-validated intervention for PTSD. Typical PE treatment is completed in 8 to 15 sessions on a weekly basis. These sessions typically last for 60 to 90 minutes. The main goal of this therapy is to directly address trauma memory and confront trauma triggers until distress decreases.

Trauma-Focused Cognitive Behavioral Therapy (TF-CBT) is an exposure therapy used for children and adolescents. This treatment is similar to PE Therapy, in which

»

children and adolescents provide a narrative of the trauma memory and process the trauma memory. It is well documented that TF-CBT is recommended as the first-line treatment for PTSD in children and adolescents.

Cognitive Processing Therapy (CPT) is typically completed in 12 weeks. The trauma survivor processes how trauma has altered their worldview (i.e., their view of self, others, and the world) and learns to challenge and modify these maladaptive thoughts. CPT teaches trauma survivors how to evaluate and change these trauma-related thoughts.

Eye Movement Desensitization and Reprocessing (EMDR) specifically targets negative emotions and focuses on using the senses, such as eye movements, hand tapping, and audio stimulation, to recover from the trauma. This treatment consists of eight phases in which processing a specific memory is completed within the first three sessions.

Non-Trauma-Focused Treatments

Stress Inoculation Therapy teaches coping skills to manage stress. This type of treatment focuses on skill training such as deep breathing, muscle relaxation, stopping negative thoughts, and restructuring or challenging maladaptive thoughts.

Acceptance and Commitment Therapy (ACT) focuses on mindfulness and acceptance. The goal of this therapy is to help a trauma survivor develop more accepting attitudes toward their distressing memories and unpleasant feelings.

Dialectical Behavior Therapy (DBT) focuses on accepting and being present in the moment (mindfulness), increasing tolerance of negative emotion (distress tolerance), changing intense emotions (emotion regulation), learning healthy ways of communicating with others, and strengthening relationships (interpersonal effectiveness). Although this treatment was originally used to help treat adults with borderline personality disorders, it has been modified to treat PTSD.

I'm Ready for Change

By opening this book, you have taken your first step in regaining control of what has been dominating your life: PTSD. Whether the title of this book sparked your interest, or the book was given to you by someone familiar with the PTSD battles you are facing, you are ready to recover and heal from trauma. Your trauma journey was not an easy one, but your road to healing and recovery will be an empowering one. At this very moment, you no longer feel trapped by your PTSD. You have shown that you no longer fear your PTSD.

Own it.

Control it.

Conquer it.

You are making the decision to move forward to a better, healthier, and positive outlook on life.

By working through this book, you will have the tools that you need to overcome PTSD. The change that you are preparing to encounter is going to take some effort, but remember, you are ready for this change because you no longer want to be "in survival mode." You want to feel alive and enjoy living in the present. PTSD no longer has to dictate your life. You have the power and control to dictate your life.

Your CBT Tool Kit

In order to regain control of your PTSD, you need to have the appropriate toolbox and tools. Not all tools will be used for the same purpose and not all tools will be used at the same time. Some tools may be sturdier than others. Some tools may have to be used more than once, and other tools may have to be combined to produce the strongest effect. You are in control and have the power to pick the tools you want to keep, the tools you want to add, and the tools you no longer need.

Think of CBT as the "toolbox" and the strategies as the "tools" that will help you overcome your PTSD. As you open this toolbox for the first time, you will be unfamiliar with what's in there. You will not know how to use the tools or when to use the tools. But as you familiarize yourself with them, you will soon learn which tool to grab to treat a specific symptom and how to use the specific tool so that life becomes easier.

Relaxation Strategies

You will grab these tools when you are experiencing hyperarousal symptoms and realize that your body is overactive. When PTSD dominates, your body's reactions rise as well. This can include an increase in blood pressure or heart rate. These reactions interfere with your ability to gain control of PTSD. These specific tools will be used to prevent or reverse strong and unhealthy physiological reactions.

Cognitive Strategies

You will grab these tools when you are experiencing intrusive thoughts. When you experience trauma and intrusive thoughts and memories, your worldview becomes distorted. These tools will help you challenge these thoughts and assess whether they are trauma-related or rational thoughts. Most importantly, these tools will be used to develop adaptive thinking patterns.

Mindfulness Strategies

You will grab these tools when you are experiencing different PTSD symptoms. PTSD can feel like you are constantly stuck in the past and worried about the future, not allowing yourself room to feel alive in the present moment. Mindfulness tools will teach you how to be present in the moment. These strategies can help remove the toxic stress linked with trauma and PTSD.

Acceptance Strategies

You will grab these tools when you feel that you have lost control over your trauma-related thoughts and emotions. These tools will help you accept your thoughts and feelings and not fight them.

Exposure Strategies

You will most likely grab these tools often, because they will come in handy when confronting your trauma triggers (e.g., avoidance symptoms). When you find yourself avoiding trauma triggers, these tools will teach you that the world is not as dangerous as you think it is.

Chapter 4 Takeaways

If you are unable to manage PTSD on your own, there is treatment available that has been studied, validated, and proven to be effective: CBT. This form of treatment is considered the "gold standard" intervention for treating PTSD. To recap, here are the main points:

- CBT is an evidence-based treatment that is proven to decrease PTSD.

- CBT specifically targets thoughts, feelings, and emotions.

- There are multiple different types of CBT intervention available.

- There are many benefits of CBT, including long-term outcomes, low relapse of symptoms, short-term therapy, and ability to regain control.

- The most well-documented and well-researched CBT intervention for PTSD is exposure therapy.

- There are multiple exposure therapies, but the most effective have been prolonged exposure therapy (for adults) and trauma-focused CBT (for children and adolescents).

- CBT offers strategies to help conquer specific PTSD symptoms.

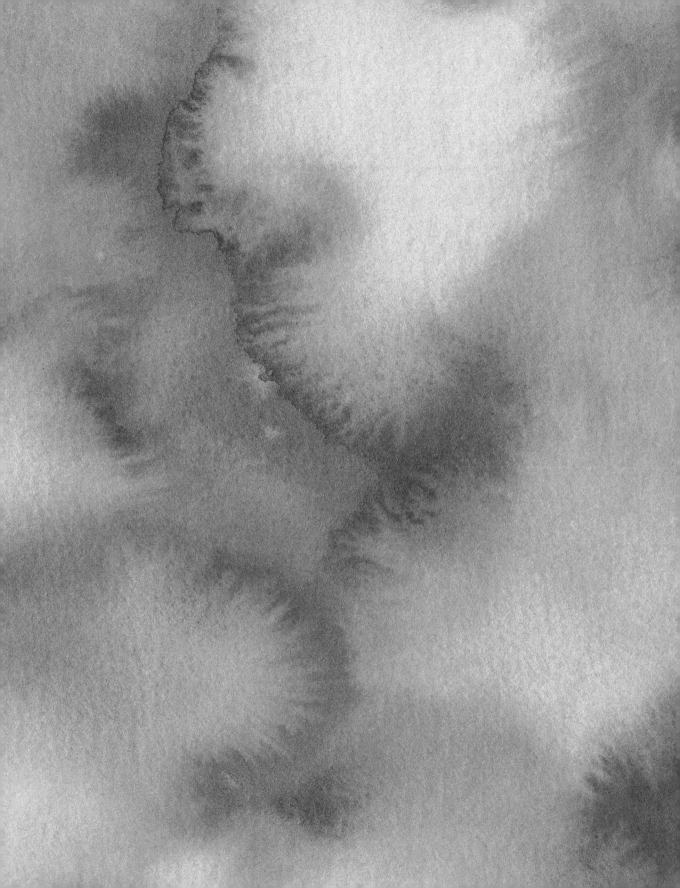

Chapter 5

Finding Your Calm

If you think about the coping strategies we talked about in chapter 1, how many are unhelpful? How many of your coping skills are relaxation strategies? This chapter will help you add relaxation strategies to your toolbox. Relaxation strategies are safe and helpful techniques that do not result in any harm to your well-being. In this chapter, you will:

- learn how stress impacts your ability to relax,

- understand the purpose of relaxation strategies,

- recognize the benefits of relaxation strategies,

- implement specific relaxation strategies,

- know how to use these relaxation strategies, and

- try these strategies yourself.

Ready? Let's go.

What Are Relaxation Strategies?

During periods of relaxation, the body experiences slower breathing, lower blood pressure, and a feeling of increased well-being. As mentioned in chapter 1 (see page 3), when you experience stress, your brain and body activate the fight-or-flight response. This releases hormones and chemicals that cause a heightened physiological response, including an increased heart rate, higher blood pressure, decreased appetite, muscle tension, and increased energy. When the stressor is resolved, your body and brain return to their baseline functioning. However, repeated exposure to chronic stress doesn't allow you to return to this relaxed baseline state.

Trauma survivors who develop PTSD may have ongoing chronic stress due to their worldview of constant fear and danger. If chronic stress persists, individuals are at risk of developing health problems such as high blood pressure, headaches, and even additional psychological disorders. Stress has also been linked to insomnia and negative emotions such as hostility, anxiety, and depression.

Benefits of Relaxation Strategies

There are numerous benefits of adding relaxation strategies to your life.

Short-term effects: Relaxation strategies can quickly reduce the physical symptoms and produce a state of calmness.

Evidence-based strategies: Relaxation strategies are a form of evidence-based treatment, meaning that studies have proven that certain relaxation strategies are effective in reducing symptoms. These strategies include progressive muscle relaxation, autogenic training, relaxation response, biofeedback, diaphragmatic breathing, guided imagery, mindfulness, and transcendental meditation.

Physical health: Research has shown that stress management techniques can treat health problems including heart disease, high blood pressure, nausea, insomnia, headaches, and chronic pain.

Depression and anxiety: Studies have found that relaxation strategies decrease symptoms of depression and anxiety. A 2019 study published in the *International Journal of Stress Management* found that when pregnant women practiced diaphragmatic breathing and progressive muscle relaxation, it lowered their stress levels and symptoms of depression.

PTSD: In a 2018 study in the *International Journal of Stress Management*, researchers found that stress inoculation decreased hyperarousal symptoms.

Alleviate Symptoms

Relaxation strategies target bodily sensations to produce the body's natural relaxation response. Although they are generally considered safe techniques, people with serious physical or psychological problems should discuss relaxation techniques with their health care providers. The goal of these techniques is to reduce the negative effects of trauma.

You have to be patient with yourself when you start applying these skills. Don't be discouraged if you are not successful on the first try. Relaxation techniques, just like any other skill, have to be learned and practiced consistently. You will get the hang of it and reap the benefits.

Deep Breathing through Imagery

Studies have shown that deep breathing can improve mood, stress, and anxiety. In order for deep breathing to be effective, it must be done correctly. The out-breath (exhale) has to be longer than the inbreath (inhale) to avoid any chance of hyperventilation. You will breathe in for 4 seconds and then out for 8 seconds.

Initially, you may find this exercise difficult, but don't be discouraged. With frequent practice, ideally daily, you will find it easier. To help determine if you are inhaling and exhaling correctly, try one of these methods:

- Lie down and place a book on your stomach to see it rise and fall with the breath.

- Place one hand on your chest and the other on your belly. The hand on your belly should rise with the inhale.

- Use a plastic straw: Inhale normally, and exhale fully through the straw.

DIRECTIONS

- Sit in a comfortable position and close your eyes, if you feel comfortable closing them. If not, just lower your gaze. With time and practice, you may allow yourself to close your eyes.

- Inhale as you count to 4, imagining smelling something that you enjoy.

- Exhale as you count to 8, imagining slowly blowing out birthday candles.

- Repeat 4 times.

Flush Away Tension
(Progressive Muscle Relaxation)

This exercise works well if you do it daily as a means of reducing tension in your body. Your body reacts by tensing up to thoughts and situations that can cause anxiety. With this exercise, as you tense and relax muscles throughout your body, you will feel an overall reduction in tension. You can use this technique whenever you start to become anxious or stressed out.

You are going to be tensing and relaxing muscles from your face all the way down to your toes. When you start to tense your muscles, it is important that you feel the tension. This may cause a bit of discomfort, but it is temporary.

You should never feel intense pain when doing this exercise. If you currently have any muscle pain or broken bones, avoid this activity until you are fully healed.

DIRECTIONS

Find a quiet, comfortable place, perhaps sitting in your car or in a room or closet in your home. You can do this exercise either sitting or lying down. The best way to engage in this exercise is with your eyes closed, but it's okay to leave your eyes open at first, if you feel uncomfortable closing them. With time and practice, you may allow yourself to close your eyes.

DEEP BREATHING

- Inhale as you count to 4, imagining smelling something that you enjoy and imagining your lungs filling.

- Exhale as you count to 8, imagining slowly blowing out birthday candles and feeling the tension leaving your body, like water flowing from a faucet.

- Practice inhaling and exhaling 3 times.

MUSCLE TENSION AND RELAXATION

While you engage in deep breathing, you will move into muscle tension and relaxation. To guide you through this exercise, use the following imagery to help with tensing muscles.

PART OF THE BODY	TENSION IMAGE
Face	Biting something sour
Jaws	Biting on a jawbreaker
Hands	Squeezing a banana
Shoulders	Raising them to the sky
Back	Touching your shoulder blades together
Stomach	Pulling your navel to your spine
Upper legs	Squeezing a balloon between your thighs
Lower legs	Pointing your toes toward you, trying to reach your head
Toes	Pushing your toes into deep sand

DIRECTIONS

1. Move your attention to your **face**. Tense the facial muscles by imagining biting something sour . . . hold it . . . 1, 2, 3, 4 . . . exhale slowly . . . feel the relaxation . . . like water flowing from a faucet. Notice the relaxation in your face. Notice it for five seconds. This is relaxation.

2. Move your attention to your **jaws**. Tense these muscles as if you were biting on a jawbreaker . . . hold it . . . 1, 2, 3, 4 . . . exhale slowly . . . feel the relaxation . . . like water flowing from a faucet. Notice the relaxation in your jaws. Notice it for five seconds. This is relaxation.

3. Move your attention to your **hands**. Tense these muscles as if you were trying to squeeze a banana . . . hold it . . . 1, 2, 3, 4 . . . exhale slowly . . . feel the relaxation . . . like water flowing from a faucet. Notice the relaxation in your hands. Notice it for five seconds. This is relaxation.

4. Move your attention to **your shoulders**. Tense these muscles as if you were trying to reach the sky with your shoulders . . . hold it . . . 1, 2, 3, 4 . . . exhale slowly . . . feel the relaxation . . . like water flowing from a faucet. Notice the relaxation in your shoulders. Notice it for five seconds. This is relaxation.

5. Move your attention to your **back**. Tense these muscles by pushing your shoulders down and back . . . hold it . . . 1, 2, 3, 4 . . . exhale slowly . . . feel the relaxation . . . like water flowing from a faucet. Notice the relaxation in your back. Notice it for five seconds. This is relaxation.

6. Move your attention to your **stomach**. Tense these muscles as if you were pulling your navel to your spine . . . hold it . . . 1, 2, 3, 4 . . . exhale slowly . . . feel the relaxation . . . like water flowing from a faucet. Notice the relaxation in your stomach. Notice it for five seconds. This is relaxation.

7. Move your attention to your **upper legs**. Tense these muscles as if you had a balloon between your thighs and are trying to pop it with your thighs . . . hold it . . . 1, 2, 3, 4 . . . exhale slowly . . . feel the relaxation . . . like water flowing from a faucet. Notice the relaxation in your upper legs. Notice it for five seconds. This is relaxation.

8. Move your attention to your **lower legs**. Tense these muscles and point your toes toward you as if you were trying to reach your head . . . hold it . . . 1, 2, 3, 4 . . . exhale slowly . . . feel the relaxation . . . like water flowing from a faucet. Notice the relaxation in your lower legs. Notice it for five seconds. This is relaxation.

9. Move your attention to your **toes**. Tense these muscles as if you were on the beach and placing your toes deep in the sand . . . hold it . . . 1, 2, 3, 4 . . . exhale slowly . . . feel the relaxation . . . like water flowing from a faucet. Notice the relaxation in your lower legs and toes. Notice it for five seconds. This is relaxation.

10. Finally, tense your **entire body** . . . face . . . jaws . . . hands and arms . . . shoulders . . . stomach . . . upper thighs . . . lower legs . . . and toes . . . tense harder . . . 1, 2, 3, 4 . . . relax . . . notice the difference . . . notice the tension . . . and notice the relaxation, like water flowing out of a faucet . . . this is relaxation. Open your eyes.

11. You are now able to distinguish the difference between tense muscles and relaxed muscles.

My Painted Safe Place (Guided Imagery)

Guided imagery is a relaxation technique that draws on your ability to visualize and daydream. This specific technique is a quick and easy relaxation strategy. Studies have demonstrated that guided imagery can reduce emotional stress and may be most effective at reducing heart rate when levels of perceived stress are low.

This exercise should help your body experience relaxation by letting your mind take you to a healthy place. The amazing thing is that you can use this relaxation exercise any time, in any given moment, in any location. Whether you are in an airplane that is about to take off or you just had a verbal disagreement with a friend, you can use this tool to help return you to a state of calmness.

DIRECTIONS

Take yourself to a place of comfort and peace in your mind. This can be anywhere you want in your city, in your state, in the country, or in the world. It can be the past, present, or future. This is going to be your painted safe place.

What place is this?

The next step is to vividly imagine the place. Before you do, look at this example for inspiration on how to paint a clearer picture of it.

PLACE	Example: *the beach*
WHAT DO YOU SEE?	*Just me, clear blue sky, the sun shining on the ocean, palm trees surrounding the golden sand, me on a secluded island, clear blue water, beautiful fish swimming near me*
WHAT DO YOU HEAR?	*Waves hitting land, birds chirping, peace, silence*
WHAT DO YOU TASTE?	*The pineapple from the tree*
WHAT DO YOU SMELL?	*Nature, clean air, the fresh air after rain*
WHAT DO THINGS THAT YOU CAN TOUCH FEEL LIKE?	*The water feels transparent, the sand feels soft, the sun hitting my skin feels hot, the flowers feel light like a feather*

Using the example in the table, describe your place in as much detail as possible.

_____

_____

_____

_____

_____

Now, make sure that you are in a comfortable position. Close your eyes. Focus on your heartbeat.

- Is it fast?

- Is it slow?

- Is it skipping beats?

- Can you imagine hearing the sound of your heartbeat?

Now, take a deep breath . . . inhale (imagine smelling something you enjoy) . . . 1 . . . 2 . . . 3 . . . 4 . . . and exhale slowly (imagine blowing out birthday candles slowly) . . . 1 . . . 2 . . . 3 . . . 4 . . . 5 . . . 6 . . . 7 . . . 8.

As you engage in deep breathing, take your mind to your comfortable, peaceful place and paint a vivid picture of what you just wrote.

- Imagine what you are seeing.

- Imagine what you are hearing.

- Imagine what you are tasting.

- Imagine what you are smelling.

- Imagine the things you touch and what they feel like.

Enjoy where you are in the present moment. Focus on how it is a stress-free place. Focus on what your body is feeling.

When you are ready to come back to reality, count backward from 10.

When you get back to the present moment, tell yourself that you feel calmer and refreshed.

Helpful Self-Talk

Self-talk is something that we all engage in. For some, this self-talk might be negative and may result in negative consequences. During stressful situations, individuals who use negative self-talk (e.g., my heart is pounding) may develop an increase in physiological arousal as the statement itself encourages the brain and body to continue activating organs and chemicals during the stressful situation. Increased negative self-talk is going to increase body stress activity.

Practicing positive self-talk during stressful situations allows your body and brain to recognize that you are not in a dangerous or harmful situation. The body and brain will work their way back to baseline functioning. The goal of this exercise is to help your body recognize that it does not need to accelerate if the situation is realistically safe and unharmful.

NEGATIVE SELF-TALK	POSITIVE SELF-TALK
I'm hyperventilating	I'm going to be okay
My heart is pounding	My body is telling me I am not relaxed
I don't like feeling this way	I know this is a natural stress response
I feel my blood pressure rising	I know that this will fade away
I'm experiencing rapid breathing	I know that I am getting enough air
I'm trembling/shaking	I know that I am not in danger

Scavenger Hunt Walk (Grounding)

Going for a walk is a great way to de-stress, if you can avoid continuing to think about your problems during the walk. Grounding techniques can help you step away from negative thoughts and come back to the present. This technique will help you distract yourself with your senses, resulting in a decrease in the intensity of your emotional reaction and negative thoughts. As you walk, scan the environment for the following:

- What are five things you hear?
- What are four things you smell?
- What are three things you can touch?
- What are two things you see?
- What is one thing you taste?

Relaxation Reflection

1. Which relaxation technique did you practice?

    ....

2. What symptoms did you alleviate?

    ....

    ....

    ....

    ....

3. How did your body feel before and after the exercise?

    ....

    ....

    ....

    ....

4. Why is it important to practice relaxation exercises?

    ....

    ....

    ....

    ....

Chapter 5 Takeaways

In this chapter you were introduced to your first set of tools. Remember, not all the tools have to be used. You may find one tool that works better for you than another tool. To recap, here are the main points:

- Your body undergoes physiological changes during stressful situations.

- Relaxation exercises target the physiological symptoms to produce the body's natural relaxation response.

- Relaxation strategies are a form of evidence-based practice.

- There are many benefits of using relaxation strategies, including quick effects and treating physiological symptoms of mental health disorders.

- Studies have shown that relaxation strategies can decrease hyperarousal symptoms in PTSD.

- There are various different types of relaxation strategies.

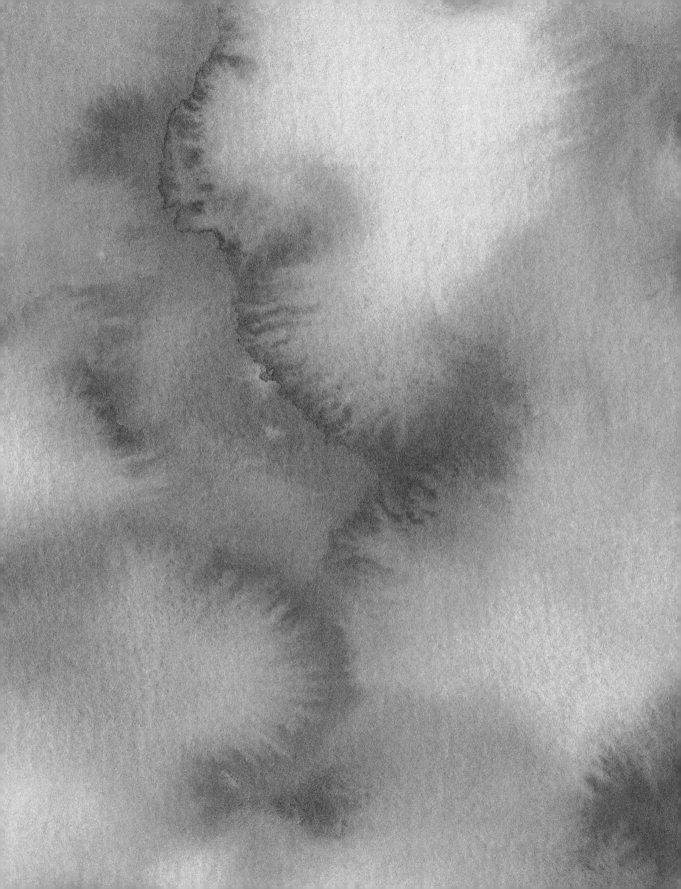

Chapter 6

Reframing Your Thoughts

You have a choice in how you respond to your trauma-related thoughts, and you have the choice of letting go of these unhealthy thoughts. In this chapter you will learn how to add healthy thinking tools to your toolbox. These specific tools will be used to help you with cognitive distortions. In this chapter, you will:

- learn about the different types of cognitive distortions,

- identify cognitive distortions,

- recognize that cognitive distortions can develop in other psychological disorders,

- become familiar with different techniques available to challenge the cognitive distortions,

- add new tools to your toolbox, and

- use more than one strategy to reframe your thoughts.

   Ready? Let's go.

What Are Cognitive Distortions?

Cognitive distortions are the central focus of cognitive behavioral therapy (CBT). Some research suggests that people develop cognitive distortions as a way of coping with negative life events. Although distorted thinking can temporarily alleviate distress, if someone is exposed repeatedly to a stressful experience, their distorted thinking can become a regular part of their daily thoughts.

One of the goals of CBT is to target these cognitive distortions. However, it's important to be able to recognize these cognitive distortions so that you can use the correct tool to challenge these faulty thoughts when they arise. Although there are multiple different kinds of cognitive distortions, researchers have identified the following as the most common thinking errors:

COGNITIVE DISTORTION	DEFINITION	EXAMPLES
Black-or-white thinking	Viewing a situation as two extremes instead of on a continuum	I'm a failure I'm not smart Nobody likes me I never do a good enough job Missing a workout routine and then saying, "I've blown my workout regimen completely."
Overgeneralization	Making incorrect broad interpretations out of a single event	Getting a low score on a math test and concluding that you are not good at math
Catastrophizing	Making negative predictions about the future, often leading to worst-case outcomes; not considering alternative outcomes	My partner didn't answer the phone, so that must mean something terrible happened

Disqualifying the positive	Recognizing the negative and ignoring the positive things that have happened	I just got lucky
Emotional reasoning	Focusing on the feeling as the truth, discounting the evidence	I feel jealous, so that means my partner is cheating on me
Labeling	Putting a fixed global label on yourself or others	He's no good I'm a loser
Magnification of negative /minimization of positive	Blowing things out of proportion and putting less weight on the positive	Mistakes are more important than progress
Mental filter	Paying attention to one negative detail exclusively instead of seeing the whole picture	I may have won first place many times, but I can't stop thinking about the one time I got second place
Mind reading	Assuming you know what others are thinking, without adequate evidence	He thinks I'm stupid She wouldn't look at me in the hallway; she probably thinks I'm ugly
Personalization	Taking things personally when events are not caused by you	It was my fault I was raped
"Should" and "must" statements	Not meeting your expectations	I should have done something I should always be friendly I should have protected my child
Tunnel vision	Only seeing the negative aspects of a situation	He just can't do anything right

Although these cognitive distortions may feel permanent, they are not. They can be corrected over time through cognitive restructuring. In simple terms, the therapist helps the patient identify and recognize the thinking error and helps the patient restructure the thought, a term referred to as cognitive reframing or restructuring.

Trauma survivors are likely to use overgeneralization due to numerous cues related to trauma triggers. That is, the maladaptive fear or fears that developed after the traumatic event start to spread across harmless cues such as certain people, places, and situations. As such, overgeneralization becomes an adaptive response to protect the trauma survivor from danger.

Research has shown that undergoing cognitive restructuring can reduce PTSD symptoms.

Alleviate Symptoms

The following exercises are strategies to help you reframe your thoughts. Be patient with yourself. Practice will help you master these skills. Remember, these strategies are not designed to treat your PTSD but to help you regain control of your trauma-related thoughts.

Check Your Thoughts

Rational thoughts are made up of known facts and are self-helpful. If we are unable to develop rational thoughts, our thoughts become maladaptive and irrational. This type of thinking is self-harming and can become a part of daily thoughts. Use the following checklist to help you determine if your thoughts are rational or irrational.

	YES	NO
Am I basing my thought on facts?		
Am I basing my thought on feelings?		
Can I see alternative solutions to my thought?		
Do other people believe the same thing that I believe?		
Do I have more than one piece of evidence to support my thought?		

Could I be misinterpreting the evidence?		
Am I confusing a fact with an opinion?		
Have I had this thought more than once?		
Has this thought become part of my daily thoughts?		
Is it hard for me to let go of this thought?		
Has this thought been self-helpful?		
Has this thought been self-harming?		

If you checked no to most of these answers, your thought is probably maladaptive. By learning that the thought is maladaptive, you can take steps to change the thought into adaptive and healthy thinking.

Weighing My Thoughts

You can use this exercise to help you determine if your thought is a fact or if your thought is an assumption, and therefore an irrational thought. The goal of this exercise is to teach you how to identify your thought as a fact or an assumption.

The body of the scale is going to be your "thought." On the left side of the scale, write down facts that make the thought true. On the right side of the scale, write down facts that make the thought false. Here is an example:

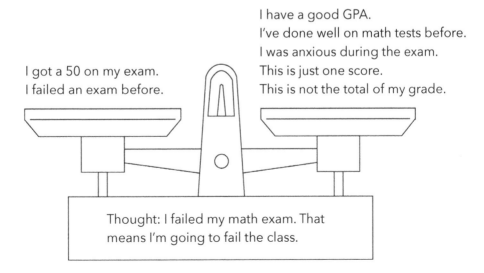

I have a good GPA.
I've done well on math tests before.
I was anxious during the exam.
This is just one score.
This is not the total of my grade.

I got a 50 on my exam.
I failed an exam before.

Thought: I failed my math exam. That means I'm going to fail the class.

Now, use the scale below to examine which side weighs more. If you have more statements on the left side, your thought is a fact. If you have more statements on the right side, your thought is false and is an assumption. As you can see in the example, there are more facts on the right side, and you can conclude that my thought is only an assumption because I have more evidence against that thought.

Now, write your thought and the facts that make it true and false on this scale.

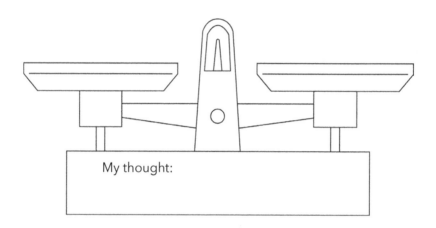

My thought:

Self-Reflection of Thought

Emotions and thoughts influence each other, and it becomes difficult to separate the two. A thought is an idea, opinion, or belief, whereas an emotion is a specific feeling, such as irritable, angry, mad, exhausted, surprised, scared, or sad.

Sometimes emotions can become more powerful than thoughts because the emotion does not match the situation or thought. For example, someone who feels angry would have thoughts related to threats (e.g., it was my fault I was abused), whereas someone who is sad would have thoughts related to loss (e.g., my boyfriend broke up with me). Someone who is feeling exhausted would have thoughts related to that specific situation (e.g., I worked a long shift today).

The goal of this exercise is to help you take a good look at your thoughts to help you examine your thoughts and identify errors that contribute to the thoughts.

MY THOUGHT	Example: *This always happens to me*	
WHAT TRIGGERED THE THOUGHT?	*I found out some bad news today*	
HOW DID IT MAKE ME FEEL? (EMOTION)	*Angry*	
HOW TRUE IS THIS THOUGHT TO ME? (0% TO 100%)	*100%*	
DOES THE THOUGHT MATCH THE EMOTION?	*No*	
HOW LIKELY IS THE THOUGHT TRUE TO OTHERS?	*20%*	
WHAT CAUSED ME TO THINK THIS WAY?	*I have a lot of bad things happen to me*	
IS THIS THOUGHT HELPFUL?	*No*	
IS THERE ANY ADVANTAGE TO MY THOUGHT?	*No*	
CAN I CONCLUDE THAT THIS THOUGHT IS AN ASSUMPTION?	*Yes*	

By completing this exercise, you should be able to notice the association between your automatic thought, emotion, and situation, and whether the thought is helpful to your well-being.

Alternative Pie Explanation

The purpose of this exercise is to help you identify your cognitive distortion and recognize that there are alternative explanations to your thought.

DIRECTIONS

1. Identify the cognitive distortion.

2. Come up with a list of possible alternative explanations related to your cognitive distortion.

3. Assign a percentage to each alternative explanation based on how likely it contributed to the thought.

4. Draw a pie chart.

5. By seeing alternatives to your thought, you can recognize that there are alternative outcomes to your thought.

Example

Automatic thought: *I failed my math test, which means I'm not smart.*

Alternative explanations

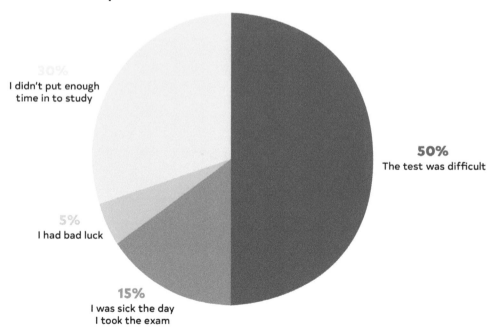

In this example, you can recognize that most likely you failed the exam because it was difficult, and not because you aren't smart enough.

Your turn:

Automatic thought: ....

....

....

Alternative explanations: ....

....

....

....

....

Pie chart:

Having a visual of the pie chart can help you recognize that there are possible alternative solutions.

(This technique is adapted from Cognitive Behavior Therapy, 2nd edition, *by Judith S. Beck.)*

STOP the Thought

Here is an acronym that you can use to help you conquer negative thoughts. Any time you have a negative thought, you can refer to "STOP" as a reminder to interfere with the maladaptive thought before it perpetuates.

Say your thought aloud

Take a second to recognize it as cognitive distortion

Objectively evaluate your thought

Prioritize the new thought

Recognize the Connection between Thoughts, Feelings, and Behaviors

There is a connection between our thoughts, feelings, and behaviors. If we can understand how all three components are interconnected, we can understand how they influence each other and reflect on how to change the thought to more adaptive functioning.

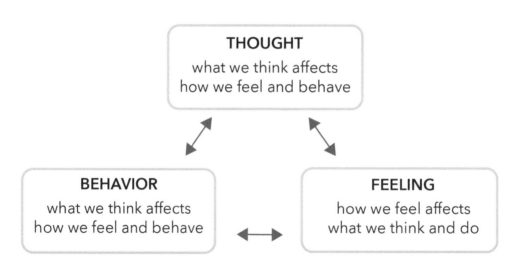

Situation: You are walking in the school hallway and the boy you like passes by you without looking.

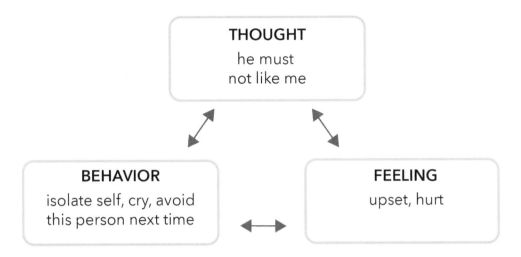

However, if you can use the tools to change the thought to an adaptive thought, your emotion and behavior will also change.

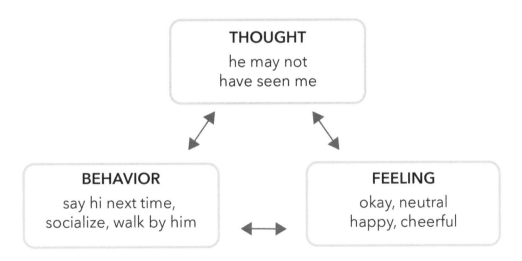

Try thinking of a recent situation that brought up negative or automatic thoughts. Look at what your thoughts, feelings, and behaviors were at that time. How might the behavior look different if you changed the thought? Write down your responses in the boxes.

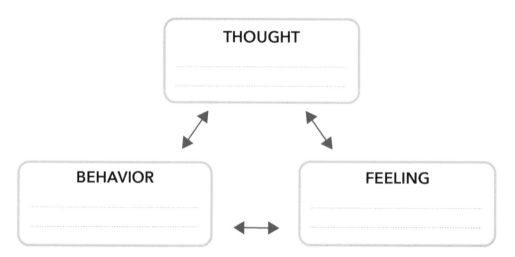

Challenge a Belief

Our beliefs capture our fundamental assumptions about the world. These beliefs are shaped by our experiences. When good things happen, we tend to have good thoughts. These thoughts are not harmful to us. However, we tend to believe bad things about ourselves and the world when bad things happen to us. This negative thinking pattern tends to hurt us more than help us. Here is a reflective exercise that can help you recognize how your old belief can negatively impact your life and how changing this belief can also change your life.

1.   My current belief about the trauma (e.g., I feel like a fraud because of my trauma):

_____

_____

_____

_____

2. How has this belief impacted my life (e.g., I stopped believing in myself; it has been difficult for me to fit in with others; I stopped making friends)?

_____

_____

_____

_____

3. A more functional or realistic belief that I can replace my current belief with is (e.g., what happened to me is not my fault):

_____

_____

_____

_____

4. How might this new belief change my life?

_____

_____

_____

_____

This exercise should help you recognize that your maladaptive thoughts have impacted your life negatively. However, if you allow yourself to change your thinking pattern, there will be a change in your life.

Reframing Thoughts Reflection

1.   Which thought-reframing technique did you practice?

2.   What symptoms did you alleviate?

3.   How did your body feel before and after the exercise?

4.   Why is it important to practice reframing your thoughts?

Chapter 6 Takeaways

This chapter provided you with tools that can help you with maladaptive thinking patterns. Remember, not all the tools have to be used. You may find that one tool works better than another tool. To recap, here are the main points:

- In CBT, negative thoughts are referred to as cognitive distortions.

- There are many common cognitive distortions (e.g., black-or-white thinking).

- Cognitive distortions are not permanent.

- Studies have shown that overgeneralization is the most common thinking error in individuals diagnosed with PTSD.

- Cognitive restructuring, which is a CBT technique, has been shown to improve symptoms of PTSD and other mental health diagnoses.

- There are multiple tools that you can use to restructure your automatic thoughts.

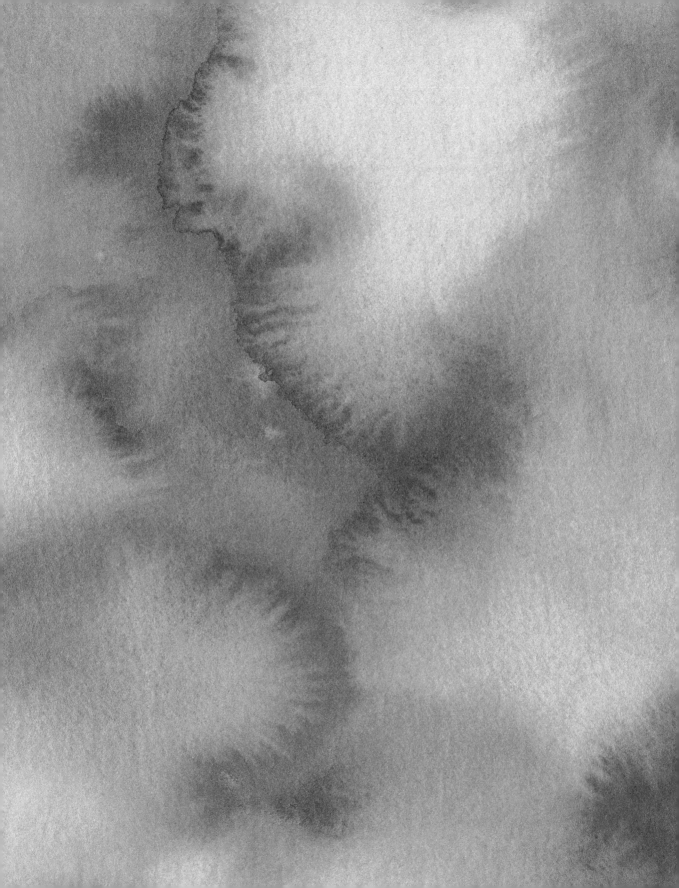

Chapter 7

Being Present, Being in the Now

Do you find yourself frequently distracted? Does your mind wander? Is it hard to remain present in the moment? With the pace at which we live, it can be difficult to slow down and be in the present moment. Mindfulness is a strategy that can teach you how to be fully present in the moment with whatever you are doing. In this chapter, you will:

- learn about mindfulness,

- understand how mindfulness impacts brain changes related to PTSD,

- know the benefits of mindfulness,

- teach yourself different mindfulness exercises, and

- add mindfulness tools to your toolbox.

   Ready? Let's go.

What Are Mindfulness Strategies?

In today's fast-paced world, how many times do you pause for a second and pay attention to the present moment? We tend to operate on autopilot during our daily experiences and we don't allow ourselves to be purposefully present in the moment. Being on autopilot all the time can become demanding on the body and mind.

Meditation is a skill that promotes well-being of the body and mind, and can help you thrive in this busy world. Think of meditation as an umbrella term and mindfulness as a form of meditation. Mindfulness focuses on these strategies:

Attention monitoring: This refers to ongoing awareness of the present moment using all the senses.

Acceptance: This refers to "welcoming in" a new perspective without judgment.

Remember, mindfulness meditation is not about becoming a different person, but training yourself to fully engage in whatever you are doing.

How Does Mindfulness Work?

Your brain uses specific pathways to process stress. As we have learned, the prefrontal cortex and amygdala are two areas of the brain that are rewired after traumatic experiences. Both of these regions play a role in fear response, while the amygdala also plays a significant role in emotion and activation of the fight-or-flight response. A 2014 study published in the journal *Current Directions in Psychological Science* found that adopting mindfulness exercises can change how the prefrontal cortex and amygdala respond to stress. Both of these areas of the brain become strengthened and more regulated with a mindfulness practice. The prefrontal cortex has more brain activity, whereas the amygdala has decreased activity. This allows you to:

• easily access your thinking and planning,

• deal with emotions during a stressful event, and

• not engage using past trauma survival mechanisms.

As you learned in chapter 3 (see page 21), avoidance is one of the core symptoms of PTSD. Research suggests that mindfulness can help reduce avoidance symptoms. Using mindfulness in conjunction with other treatments or strategies can help trauma survivors bring awareness to their thoughts and feelings surrounding the traumatic event, instead of avoiding them.

What Are the Benefits of Mindfulness?

Mindfulness practices have been incorporated into several mental health thera-pies, including mindfulness-based stress reduction, mindfulness-based cognitive therapy, dialectical behavior therapy, and acceptance and commitment therapy. All these therapies are useful in treating PTSD and have resulted in:

- reduction in avoidance symptoms,

- improvement in shame-based beliefs, and

- improvement in self-blame thoughts.

   Research has shown that mindfulness strategies improve the psychological and physical well-being of individuals. Mindfulness techniques have also resulted in multiple benefits to individuals:

Reduced PTSD symptoms: Studies have found that individuals who practice mindfulness skills reported lower levels of PTSD symptoms, better regulation of their emotions, and a reduction in avoidance symptoms.

Reduced depression and anxiety: Mindfulness can help alleviate depression and anxiety, especially recurring negative thinking. Mindfulness can also be effec-tive in preventing relapses of depression.

Improved physical well-being: Studies have shown that mindfulness decreases blood pressure and improves immune function.

Improved emotional regulation: Mindfulness training can help individuals become more aware of their emotions, as well as regulate their emotions.

Improved quality of life: Mindfulness-based interventions can improve general well-being for many individuals. For example, these techniques have improved quality of life for individuals diagnosed with chronic pain, cancer patients, and individuals diagnosed with a variety of mental disorders, including anxiety.

Alleviate Symptoms

PTSD survivors frequently find themselves stuck in the past because of intrusive thoughts and flashbacks, while also worrying about the future because of per-ceived trauma-related fears. Because of this, trauma survivors are unable to be fully present in the moment. These mindfulness exercises will help you during challenging and stressful times. These exercises are not going to alleviate all your PTSD symptoms, but they will help you be present in the moment.

Present in the Current Situation

One trauma trigger may cause a flashback or intrusive thought. One trauma trigger may cause poor emotional control. One trauma trigger may impact the rest of your day. When trauma survivors experience an intrusive thought or flashback, their concentration becomes impaired and they are not present in the moment. When you are experiencing a flashback or intrusive thought, use this exercise to help bring yourself back into the present moment.

DIRECTIONS

Whatever room you are in, pick one object to focus on. This can be anything from a lamp to the sofa you are sitting on to the clock on the wall. Focus on the specific object and use your imagination and five senses to describe the object.

Sight: What does the object look like? Do you see any shapes? Do you see any colors? Do you see any patterns?

Sound: What might the object sound like if you touch it? What might the object sound like if you drop it? What might the object sound like if you shake it?

Smell: Does the object have any particular old smell? Does the object have any particular new smell? Does the object have a particular odor?

Taste: How might the object taste? Hard? Soft? How many bites would it take? How might it feel on your teeth?

Touch: How does this object feel? Is it soft? Is it hard? Is it bumpy? Is the object heavy?

Be Mindful of Your Body

The purpose of this exercise is for you to notice your bodily sensations and become aware of them in the present moment.

DIRECTIONS

Pay attention to your body right now, in this moment. Write down what is happening with your body (e.g., I have pain that stings in my lower back; the muscles in my neck are tense; my hands feel cold).

....

....

....

When you think about your trauma, pay attention to your body. What is your body experiencing in the moment? What is happening to your body (e.g., my body shakes when I think about my trauma; my cheeks start to turn red; my heart skips a beat; there is a lump in my throat)?

....

....

....

Begin deep breathing (see page 62). You can also engage in an imagery exercise by imagining something that you enjoy smelling (inhale) and slowly blowing out birthday candles (exhale). Remember to make your inhale shorter than your exhale. Repeat three times.

Pay attention to your breathing. Is it slow? Is it fast?

Pay attention to your heartbeat. Is it slow? Is it fast?

Keep practicing deep breathing.

If you find yourself drifting off with your thoughts, it's okay. Bring yourself back to the present moment by focusing on your physical symptoms.

Pay attention to your face, hands, arms, stomach, legs, toes.

If your thoughts wander off, bring them back to focus on your body.

Relax.

Pay attention to your body after this exercise. What do you notice (e.g., my heart beat slowed down; my hands became warm)?

....

....

....

Labeling Your Emotions

Trauma survivors often avoid or escape unpleasant emotions because they are typically viewed as being harmful. Trauma survivors will also use phrases to explain their emotions without labeling the actual emotion itself. By bringing mindful awareness to your emotions, you can notice the emotion, accept it, not fear it or struggle against it, and label it. In the following table are some helpful phrases that you can use to label your emotions.

TRAUMA-RELATED EMOTIONAL RESPONSE	PRESENT MOMENT EMOTIONS
I don't need to talk about my trauma	Fear (I feel nervous because I do not want to talk about my trauma)
I want to punch the wall right now	Anger (I'm angry because what you said reminded me of my trauma)
I've moved on from my past	Fear (It is okay to feel scared because I was hurt)
You can't tell me how I should be feeling	Relief (Thanks for recognizing that right now I do not feel like myself)
I want to cry right now but I can't	Sadness (It's okay to feel sad; sadness is a normal feeling)
It's easier to forget what happened to me	Confusion (I feel confused because of what happened to me)

Following the example just given, use the next table to create your own trauma-related emotional responses, and labels.

WHAT IS YOUR TRAUMA-RELATED EMOTIONAL RESPONSE?	GIVE THE TRAUMA-RELATED EMOTIONAL RESPONSE A LABEL

Daily Mindfulness Activity

There are many opportunities throughout the day to practice mindfulness. Pick an activity that you engage in daily. It could be brushing your teeth, taking a shower, eating breakfast, walking, gardening, riding the subway, reading, etc. Whatever the activity, allow yourself five minutes to pay attention. Focus your attention on the sensations of the activity. As you become familiar with this exercise, look for opportunities throughout your day to be more mindful.

For example, the next time you're gardening, be present in the moment by focusing on what you are doing. Feel the warm sun hitting your back as you lean over to pull out the weeds. Enjoy the warmth of the outdoor weather. Listen to the neighbor next door mowing their grass. Pay attention to how the sunflower seed has blossomed into a tall sunflower. Feel how cold the water is when you water your garden.

Emotional Company

This exercise will help you become aware of whatever emotions show up. You have the right to experience a full range of emotional responses. Whatever emotion you are experiencing is valid. Emotions are going to come, whether or not you want them to. We tend to keep the "positive" emotions company but find ways to escape the "negative" emotions. The next time a negative emotion joins you, allow it to be in your company. Allow yourself to feel the emotion for as long as you need. Become familiar with these emotions. Start to recognize these emotions.

Ask yourself:

1. What does this emotion need?
2. What is this emotion afraid of?
3. What would make it better?
4. How would this emotion feel if the problem were gone?
5. What is this emotion telling me?
6. Is this emotion helping me?
7. Is this emotion hurting me?
8. How long has this emotion been hanging around for?
9. Can this emotion hang around?
10. Can I survive this emotion?

Allow this emotion to help you recognize that you are experiencing a moment of suffering.

Being Mindful of Your Thoughts

When we give meaning to our thoughts, the thoughts have a big impact on how our day unfolds. We start to evaluate the thought, make assumptions about the thought, and spend a lot of time fixating on the thought. Thoughts often lead to physical sensations, which can include rapid heart rate, sweatiness, and increased blood pressure. As long as you continue to judge your thoughts, the sensations will continue. If you judge your thoughts, you will also judge your bodily sensations. Physical sensations are normal; they help us function and they do not have to feel dangerous. We can choose to not judge our thoughts, and then the sensations will pass.

The goal of this exercise is to help you become mindful of your thoughts and recognize that if you do not judge your thoughts, the bodily sensations will subside.

DIRECTIONS

Pay attention to your current thoughts. Write down these thoughts without judgment.

_____

_____

_____

Now think about your trauma and write down your reaction (e.g., my body shakes when I think about my trauma; my cheeks start to turn red; my heart skips a beat; there is a lump in my throat).

_____

_____

_____

All these thoughts, whether trauma related or not, are just that, thoughts. They are not permanent, and they will eventually pass. When we pay attention to our thoughts, we can choose to not judge them or give them meaning. When we do not judge our thoughts, our bodily sensations remain stable. When we start to give meaning to our thoughts, bodily sensations increase. Allow these thoughts to be present, but choose to not judge them.

Chapter 7 Takeaways

Mindfulness is a beneficial tool that can be used to help you recognize that you are living a more mindful life; that is, being fully present in the moment more often. To recap, here are the main points:

- Mindfulness is a form of meditation that promotes well-being of the body and mind.

- Mindfulness is used in evidence-based treatments.

- Mindfulness can treat symptoms of PTSD.

- This skill can be practiced on a daily basis.

- With mindfulness you use your five senses to be present without judgment.

- There are various mindfulness strategies that can be used.

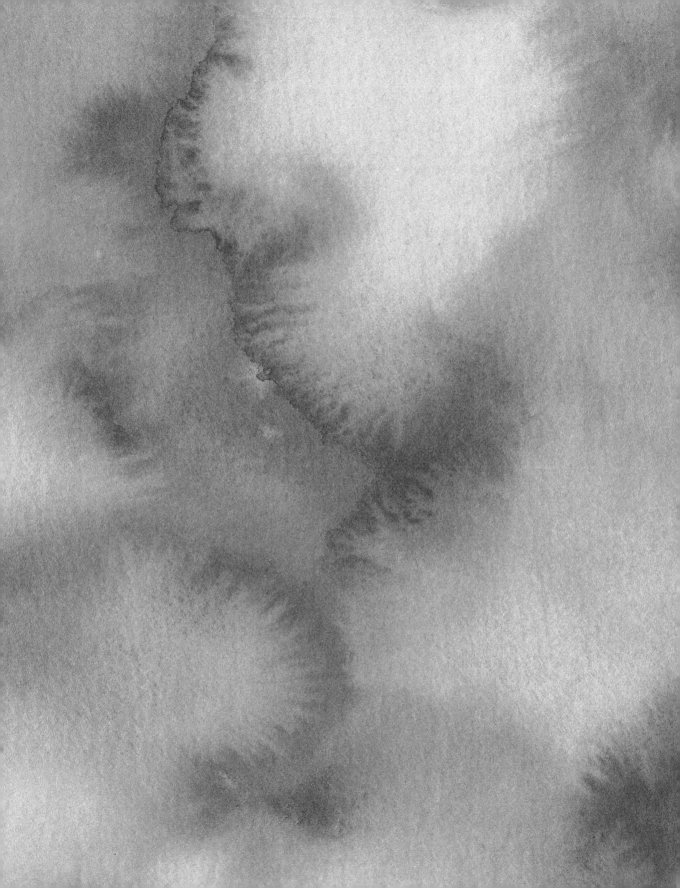

Chapter 8

Learning to Accept the Uncertain

How many times have you tried to stop your intrusive thoughts? How many times have you tried to avoid your emotions? Have you ever tried to allow yourself to just accept? In this chapter, you will learn about acceptance strategies that will help you embrace your thoughts and feelings and encourage you to develop a compassionate relationship with your trauma experiences. In this chapter, you will:

- learn how acceptance strategies can help a trauma survivor,

- become familiar with different acceptance exercises,

- practice acceptance strategies, and

- add these acceptance strategies to your toolbox.

Ready? Let's go.

What Are Acceptance Strategies?

Your trauma is a fact from the past, and that cannot change. However, the thoughts and emotions that developed after the trauma can be accepted into your life. The purpose of your thoughts is to help you understand your world as best you can. The purpose of your emotions is to help you survive. Thus, you cannot eliminate your thoughts and emotions. You cannot erase the traumatic memory, but you can learn how to accept the memory and the painful and unpleasant thoughts and feelings.

In order to cope, trauma survivors are likely to find strategies that help them avoid their trauma-related thoughts, feelings, and memories. For example, a trauma survivor may use alcohol to avoid the emotional pain of losing their partner to cancer. Because the trauma survivor learns that alcohol "gets rid of" the emotional pain, they continue to increase their alcohol consumption. These unhealthy coping strategies temporarily help, but have more debilitating long-term effects.

Instead of avoiding and turning to unhealthy coping strategies, there are strategies that can help you accept the uncomfortable memories, thoughts, and feelings. These strategies are used in a specific CBT treatment known as acceptance and commitment therapy (ACT). Strategies from this therapy focus on you taking a step back and observing your thinking. It can teach you how to allow yourself to experience these private events as they are, without feeling overwhelmed by them. Acceptance strategies can also help address self-criticism, self-stigma, and shame, which are common reactions reported by trauma survivors.

Accepting an emotion or thought does not mean that you are accepting what happened to you. It does not mean that you are condoning, liking, or feeling good about your trauma. Instead, you are accepting the truth of the situation (e.g., a trauma has happened to me) and allowing yourself to learn about your thinking pattern and negative emotions. Accepting thoughts and emotions for what they are allows you to become less fearful in your daily life.

Because trauma-related thoughts can become a part of daily thoughts, trauma survivors tend to view their thinking as a literal reflection of the truth. For example, a trauma survivor who thinks, "I am damaged or broken as a result of my trauma" can choose unhealthy and unhelpful ways to react to that thought, including social isolation, suicidal behavior, or poor self-image.

Acceptance strategies can help the trauma survivor:

- recognize that thoughts are just words put together and then choose to evaluate the thought and respond in a healthier way,

- create a healthier perspective about themselves and the world, and

- better control their emotions.

Research has shown that acceptance strategies are a promising treatment for PTSD. Several studies have found that trauma survivors who receive ACT have better control of their PTSD. A 2017 study published in the journal *Cognitive and Behavioral Practice* found that three participants experienced improvements in depression, anxiety, and PTSD symptoms after receiving ACT.

Alleviate Symptoms

The following exercises use acceptance strategies to help you regain control of your PTSD. By no means when you engage in these exercises are you accepting that what happened to you is okay. Rather, the goal of these exercises is to help you recognize that there is an alternative and healthier view of your trauma.

Examining Old Habits

The goal of this exercise is to help you recognize that avoiding your trauma-related thoughts and emotions has not been working. A new way of looking at things may lead to a different outcome and a new, improved way of living.

WAYS I'VE TRIED TO GET RID OF UNWANTED THOUGHTS/EMOTIONS	Example: *Drinking alcohol*	
HOW EFFECTIVE WAS THIS STRATEGY? 0 = NOT AT ALL 10 = VERY	1	
DID THIS REDUCE YOUR SYMPTOMS IN THE SHORT TERM	Yes	

»

DID IT REDUCE SYMPTOMS IN THE LONG TERM?	*No*	
DID IT BRING YOU CLOSER TO THE LIFE YOU WANT?	*No*	
WHAT DID THIS STRATEGY COST YOU? (e.g., ENERGY, HEALTH, RELATIONSHIPS)	*Getting fired from a job*	
ARE YOU OPEN TO TRYING SOMETHING DIFFERENT?	*Yes*	

ACCEPT

Use this acronym as a reminder that you can accept your thoughts and feelings just as they are, without having to change them or use unhealthy ways to cope with them.

Accept thoughts and emotions as part of life

Choose to not avoid your thoughts and emotions

Choose to have control over your thoughts and emotions

Experience the thoughts and emotions as they are

Pay attention to the present moment

Take control of your acceptance

More Accepting of My Thoughts

Acceptance means identifying your experience and simply acknowledging it rather than judging your thoughts as "bad," "trauma thoughts," or "not good thoughts." The goal of this exercise is to help you recognize that you can have healthy control over your thinking by allowing your thoughts to just remain there, without you judging them.

1. Write down a trauma-related thought.

_____

_____

_____

_____

2. How have you labeled this thought (e.g., bad thought, trauma thought, horrible thinking)?

_____

_____

_____

_____

3. What would it be like if you allowed yourself to just accept the thought as it is?

_____

_____

_____

_____

4. What would it be like if you did not judge your thought?

_____

_____

_____

_____

More Accepting of My Emotions

Similar to the previous exercise, you can identify your experience and simply acknowledge it, rather than judging your emotions as "bad feelings," "trauma feelings," or "not-so-good feelings." The goal of this exercise is to help you recognize that you can have healthy control over your symptoms by allowing your emotions to just remain there, without you reacting to them.

1.   Write down a trauma-related emotion.

_____

_____

_____

_____

2.   How have you labeled this emotion (e.g., scary, unwanted, not-so-good feelings)?

_____

_____

_____

_____

3.   What would it be like if you allowed yourself to just accept and experience the emotion?

_____

_____

_____

_____

4. What would it be like if you did not judge your emotion?

_____

_____

_____

_____

Observe Your Language

The goal of this exercise is to help you recognize how much meaning you are giving to your trauma-related thoughts and/or emotions. This exercise will help you recognize your thoughts, images, and memories as what they are–nothing more than language, words, and pictures–as opposed to what they can appear to be–threatening events, rules that must be obeyed, lies that you told yourself, etc.

1. Write down a trauma-related thought.

_____

_____

_____

_____

2. Read that thought silently three times to yourself.

3. Notice what happens to you and your body. Write down what is happening.

_____

_____

_____

_____

4. Now say that exact trauma-related thought aloud three times.

5. Notice what happens to you and your body. What is happening? Is it different from when you read the trauma-related thought silently?

_____

_____

_____

_____

6. Now replace that same thought with a new phrase: "I have the thought that . . ." Write it down (e.g., "I have the thought that I deserved the trauma").

7. Now say the new phrase three times aloud.

8. Notice what happens to you and your body. What is happening? Is it different when you change the language of your thought?

_____

_____

_____

_____

This exercise should have helped you recognize that you don't have to get rid of the thought. You can regard the thought as just words. By the end of the exercise, the thought should have less impact on you than when you started.

Give Less Meaning to Your Thoughts

1. Write down a recent trauma-related thought/emotion.

_____

_____

_____

2.   Rate your trauma-related thought/emotion based on how distressing it is (0 = not at all; 10 = very much).

0   1   2   3   4   5   6   7   8   9   10

Rate how much distress it would cause you if you saw your thought in these forms:

REFRAMING THE THOUGHT	RATE LEVEL OF DISTRESS (1 TO 10)
Imagine that the thought is just a lyric from a song	
Imagine that the thought/emotion is words on a karaoke screen	
Imagine that the thought/emotion is a sentence read from a poem	
Imagine that the thought/emotion is a subtitle in a movie you are watching	
Imagine that the thought/emotion is a text message from a family member/ friend	
Imagine that the thought/emotion is a sentence in a nonfiction book	
Imagine that the thought/emotion is a quote you read somewhere	

As you read each item of imagery, your distress should have decreased. The goal is not to get rid of these thoughts/emotions, but simply to learn how to step back and see them for what they are: just "words passing through."

Willingness to Accept My Thoughts and Emotions

The goal of this exercise is to help you take the first step in accepting your thoughts and emotions for what they are: just thoughts and emotions.

Write down 10 common trauma-related thoughts and emotions that come to your mind. Then circle the two thoughts and emotions you are willing to start to accept as just thoughts and just emotions. Whenever these two thoughts and emotions come into your mind, allow them to sit there until they pass by.

THOUGHTS	EMOTIONS

Chapter 8 Takeaways

Your trauma event has been imprinted on your brain and cannot be erased. However, you can learn to accept what happened and accept the trauma-related thoughts and emotions without trying to avoid or change them. To recap, here are the main points:

- Acceptance strategies help you experience your private events as they are.

- Studies have shown that these strategies can help alleviate symptoms of PTSD, especially avoidance symptoms.

- Acceptance strategies originated from ACT.

- Acceptance strategies are additional tools that can be added to your toolbox.

- There are different types of acceptance strategies that you can use.

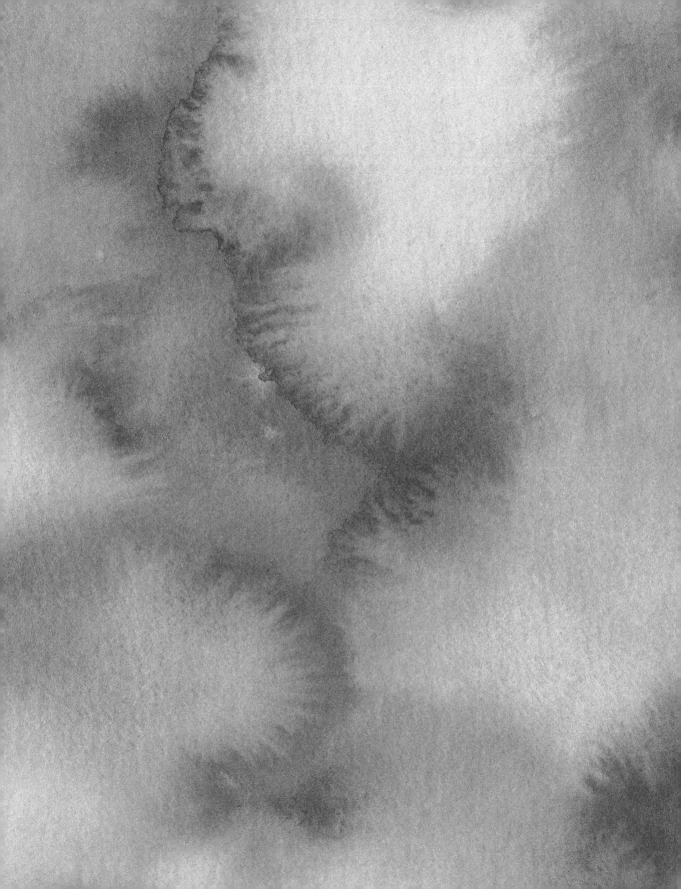

Chapter 9

Exposing Yourself to Your Fears

If you could confront your trauma-related fears, which one would you choose? Confronting your fears may seem frightening, but it doesn't have to be. Some specific exposure strategies can help you recognize and reflect on your avoidance of trauma triggers. In this chapter, you will:

- learn about two specific types of exposure strategies, imaginal exposure and *in vivo* exposure,

- gain insight about how avoidance maintains the fear,

- become familiar with the term "habituation,"

- add exposure-like strategies to your toolbox,

- reflect on your own trauma triggers, and

- understand the difference between perceived threats and actual threats.

Ready? Let's go.

What Are Exposure Strategies?

After a traumatic event has occurred, trauma survivors often avoid anything that reminds them of that experience. Although avoidance may provide temporary relief, it eventually maintains the fear and makes PTSD stick around longer.

Avoiding your fears often leads to unhealthy behavioral patterns, such as substance use, to escape the emotional pain and memories. Confronting your fears can actually be accomplished in a healthy and safe way. Imagine how empowering it will feel to conquer your trauma triggers without feeling that you are in danger.

Reducing the fear associated with trauma reminders can be accomplished through specific types of exposure. Although there are a variety of exposure strategies, here are two well-known and researched exposure strategies in the treatment of PTSD:

Imaginal exposure: Trauma survivors are asked to mentally imagine their trauma and share the details of the traumatic event.

***In vivo* exposure:** The individual directly confronts safe trauma reminders. Examples include driving by the location where the trauma happened, looking at an image of a trauma trigger, or touching an object that can trigger memories of the trauma.

Both of these exposure techniques are implemented in prolonged exposure therapy (PE). This therapy is considered the treatment of choice for PTSD because it's been shown to be effective in reducing trauma symptoms. In fact, PE is recommended worldwide in an official PTSD treatment guideline. These exposure strategies are conducted in a safe environment that allows the trauma survivor to confront the fear-related memories and trauma triggers.

As the trauma survivor is repeatedly (and safely) exposed to their memories and trauma triggers, their fear gradually decreases with each exposure. This is called habituation. This particular approach works in reducing bodily sensations, such as increased heart rate, and proves to the trauma survivor that these trauma triggers aren't actually dangerous.

Exposure strategies help trauma survivors recognize that their traumatic experience is not as dangerous as it's perceived to be. It helps them differentiate between perceived and actual life threats. Overall, exposure strategies can help the trauma survivor put on a different lens and view the world from a healthy perspective.

In chapter 4 (see page 47), you learned about emotional processing theory, which basically suggests that fear networks are formed following exposure to a traumatic event. This fear network is resistant to modification. During the habituation process, the trauma-related fear is activated, and you eventually learn that you can handle your fear.

Several studies have shown that habituation is effective in reducing PTSD symptoms, and that exposure-based strategies can decrease physiological symptoms of PTSD, including increased heart rate. In a 2019 study published in the *Journal of Psychiatric Research*, researchers found that exposure strategies helped decrease symptoms in soldiers with PTSD. The soldiers experienced the biggest change in avoidance and numbing symptoms, and when they underwent a two-week intensive PE treatment, they experienced a reduction in heart rate when reacting to trauma triggers.

Alleviate Symptoms

The following exercises are not meant to have you engage in direct imaginal and *in vivo* exposures, as these specific techniques require a trained professional to guide you through the exposures and confront the fears.

You should not experience significant distress with the following exposure strategies. The goals of these strategies are to help you recognize your fears, reflect on the severity of your fears, and gain a better understanding of how your trauma-related fears are impacting your quality of life. If you find yourself experiencing distress, do not proceed with these exercises.

Recognize Trauma Triggers as Threats

There is a difference between real threats and perceived threats. Although both share common bodily sensations (e.g., increased heart rate) and emotional reactions (e.g., fear), real threats endanger our existence whereas perceived threats cause unwarranted anxiety.

In the following chart, identify whether the following are a threat to you:

PLACES	YES	NO
The address where the trauma happened		
A Google image of the location		
The nearest street sign where the trauma happened		
Restaurants		
Bars		
Sporting events		
Specific homes		
Specific areas in a home (e.g., basement)		
Hospitals		
Parks		
PEOPLE	**YES**	**NO**
Specific people who were directly associated with your trauma		
Specific gender of the person		
Encountering someone with physical traits that remind you of someone involved in the trauma		
THINGS	**YES**	**NO**
Specific odors (list the smells)		
Specific clothing (list the clothing)		
Types of food (list the food)		
Body closeness		

People standing or sitting next to you		
Hugs		
Tone of voice		
Authority figures		
Loud noises (list the noises)		
Specific weather (e.g., rain)		
Holidays		
Nighttime		
Vehicles (e.g., cars, trucks)		
An anniversary		
An argument		
Watching a movie or show that reminds you of your traumatic event		
News articles that remind you of the traumatic event		
Specific colors		
Specific words or phrases		
Anything else not listed (list the items)		

If you checked yes to any of these items, you have identified them as threatening to you because in some way these items are your trauma triggers. Trauma survivors avoid trauma triggers because the items have been "programmed" in the brain as threatening, unsafe, harmful, or dangerous. These trauma triggers (with a few exceptions) are most likely objectively safe places, individuals, and things. When you are faced with your trauma trigger (exposure), you can start to recognize that it is a perceived threat and not an actual threat.

Recognize Perceived vs. Actual Threats

When you are triggered, you are flooded with emotions that then influence your perception and reactions. As soon as your body has identified a threat, it prepares you to respond to the identified threat. Because trauma survivors identify trauma triggers as perceived threats, a trauma trigger causes the survivors to react as if the threat were present in real time, even if it isn't. Over time, these responses become automatic and you react without awareness.

Here are examples of perceived trauma-related threats and actual threats. See if you can add any other types of threats.

PERCEIVED THREAT	ACTUAL THREAT
Memory of my trauma	Someone threatening you
Specific locations	A bear coming toward you
Specific individuals	A fire
Physical traits of people that remind me of a person connected with my trauma	Lack of oxygen
Arguments	Hurricane
Objects	Tornado
Smells	Car accident
Colors	Physical hazards
Loud noises	Chemical hazards
Anniversaries	Venomous snake
Failure	Black widow spider
Fireworks	Severe allergic reaction
Phobias	Animals that transmit disease
Leaving the house	Plants with sharp spines that can puncture skin, feet, and eyes

1. How do you react to your perceived threats?

_____

_____

_____

2. How would someone react to actual threats?

_____

_____

_____

Your Survival Instincts

To better understand how you respond to fearful situations, it's important to recognize the fight, flight, or freeze response. This response plays a critical role in you surviving truly threatening situations. However, trauma survivors with PTSD mistake their body's response to a perceived threat as an indication that there is a real threat. Understanding more about the fight, flight, or freeze response can help you be proactive with your response style and feel safer. By learning how your body reacts to stress, you can step ahead of your learned trauma reaction.

NOTICEABLE EFFECTS	HIDDEN EFFECTS	FREEZE EFFECTS
Dilated pupils	Brain prepares for action	Mind goes blank
Fast heartbeat	Food movement slows down	Emotions shut down
Chest pain	Blood pressure increases	Fainting
Pale or flushed skin	Adrenaline releases to blood	Looking dazed
Muscle tension	Heart pumps more blood	Daydreaming
More alert and observant		Freezing
Dry mouth		Dissociation
Chills		

Use the following exercise to help you recognize your survival instincts and how they impact you.

TRAUMA FEAR	Example: *Looking at a picture of the street where I was abused*	
IS MY FEAR AN ACTUAL THREAT OR PERCEIVED THREAT?	*Perceived threat*	
MY NOTICEABLE EFFECTS OF FIGHT, FLIGHT, OR FREEZE	*Fast heartbeat, muscle tension, chest pain*	
ARE MY BRAIN AND BODY RECOGNIZING THAT I AM IN DANGER?	*Yes*	
IS MY REACTION APPROPRIATE TO THE FEAR?	*No*	
WHAT WOULD BE AN APPROPRIATE REACTION TO THE FEAR?	*Just looking at the picture without feeling scared*	

Recognize When Survival Instincts Aren't Needed

Use the following diagram to help you recognize if your threat is actual or perceived. By being able to identify your threat as a "perceived threat," you can begin to control your PTSD by not activating your fight, flight, or freeze response. You will learn how to respond to your trauma triggers in a healthier way.

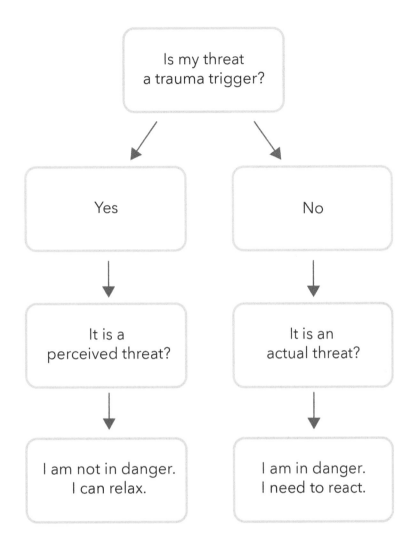

Giving Less Power to My Perceived Fears

The amount of power we give to our fears often stems from the meaning that we give to the trauma triggers. You can choose to give less power to these fears by recognizing what the purpose of the specific trauma trigger is. For example, a trauma survivor who was robbed at the park may think, "the park (trauma trigger) is dangerous (perceived fear) because I was physically injured there." The trauma survivor can choose to continue to identify "the park" as dangerous or can change the meaning to simply "the park is a place to jog, play a sport, relax, or spend time with friends."

TRAUMA TRIGGER	WHAT THE TRAUMA TRIGGER MEANS TO ME	THE ACTUAL MEANING
Example: *Yellow umbrellas*	*Yellow umbrellas are unsafe because I was holding one when I was hit by a car while crossing the street*	*Yellow umbrellas are used to protect people from rain*
Example: *Trains*	*Trains are dangerous because I was assaulted next to the train station*	*Trains are used for public transportation*

Change the Details of Your Nightmares

You cannot change the trauma that happened to you. But you can reframe the nightmares that continue to haunt you. By re-creating these nightmares, you are allowing yourself to confront them instead of using unhealthy ways to avoid having nightmares, including choosing not to sleep.

What is the worst memory of your nightmare?

....

....

....

Change the location of your nightmare. How would the nightmare be different?

....

....

Change the people in your nightmare. How would the nightmare be different?

....

....

Change some of the things in your nightmare. How would the nightmare be different?

....

....

Change the emotions in your nightmare. How would the nightmare be different?

....

....

Change the theme of the nightmare to "survived." How would the nightmare be different?

....

....

Chapter 9 Takeaways

· ·

Exposure strategies are a useful tool to help you recognize that your trauma fears are not as scary as you perceive them to be in your head. To recap, here are the main points:

- Two well-known exposure strategies are imaginal exposure and *in vivo* exposure.

- Exposure strategies are part of the well-known prolonged exposure (PE) therapy, one of the most researched evidence-based treatments.

- Diminished fear as a result of repetitive exposure is referred to as habituation.

- Studies show exposure strategies can reduce avoidance and physical symptoms in individuals with PTSD.

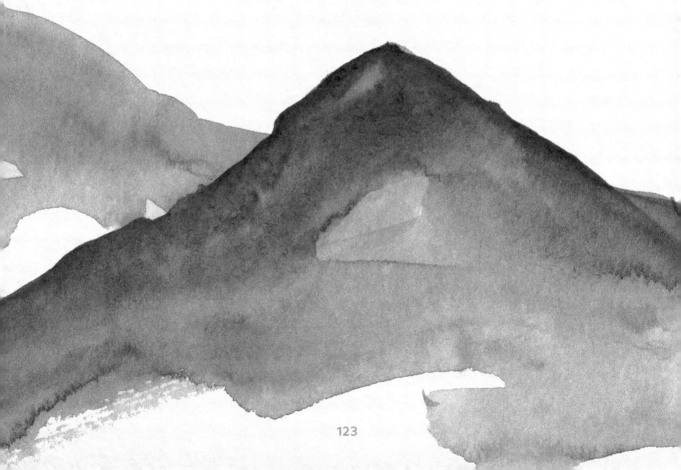

Part 3

Surviving & Thriving with PTSD

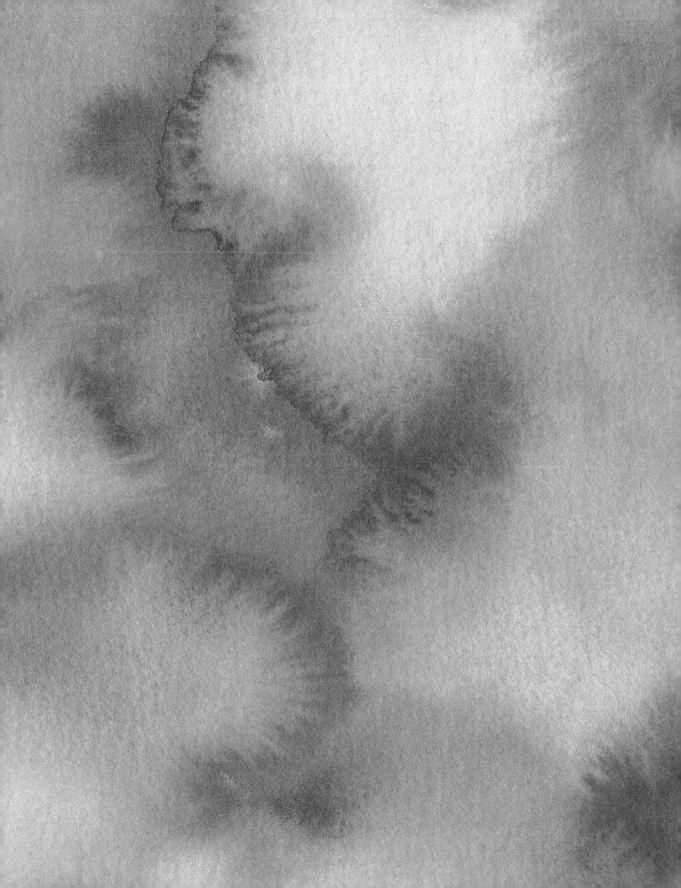

Chapter 10

Continuing to Heal

If you have gotten this far in the workbook, you most likely have found some value along your path to healing and recovery. However, you probably also realize that PTSD is an ongoing journey. In this chapter, you will:

- learn how to use a metaphor to understand your PTSD journey,

- learn about the different types of medication to treat PTSD,

- become familiar with medication-specific symptom reduction, and

- engage in an exercise to rediscover your purpose.

   Ready? Let's go.

Long-Term Outlook

Your trauma journey is personal and unique to you. Although people can walk similar paths, no one can walk the exact same path as you. As mentioned earlier, your trauma journey was not an easy one, but your road to healing and recovery is a powerful one.

You must remember that healing from PTSD is a lifelong journey of learning how to improve your quality of life on a daily basis that leads to a better and healthier you. Life in general, whether you've experienced a trauma or not, is not meant to be easy, but a continuing walk full of both hardships and triumphs.

This is your personal journey, and no one can take it away from you. Use the following metaphor as an example of your PTSD journey, the hardships that come with PTSD, and your triumphs.

For the longest time you have walked down the same path. This time, you decide to take a new path. A path that is unfamiliar to you. A path that may be uncomfortable for you. But as you continue to walk down this path, what once was unfamiliar and uncomfortable becomes familiar and comfortable.

On this path, you will run into things from your past, but you will view them with a new perspective. The trees that you once viewed as scary are no longer frightening. What was once foggy is now clear. The flowers that seemed dull are more vibrant. On this new path, you will encounter more sunny days than rainy days. You will encounter more color and more beauty. However, you have to remember that even a more alive, colorful, and beautiful path can also have unforeseen circumstances.

On your new path, you may encounter unpleasant weather conditions such as thunderstorms or hail; reminders of your old path, such as seeing the same flock of birds or similar plants; or an unforeseen circumstance such as a flood that brings you back to your pain and suffering. This flood may make you pause on your path and reconsider your direction.

Any unforeseen circumstance you encounter as you walk your path is a reminder that you have survived more difficult times; you have survived more difficult events. You cannot avoid or control the unforeseen circumstances that will come your way, but when they do come your way, they will be reminders that you can conquer anything. As the flood clears, you choose to continue pursuing this better path. You are in control of your final destination.

PTSD Medication

Because there are limited numbers of trained therapists who deliver trauma-focused psychotherapy, pharmacotherapy—or medication—has been the most readily available treatment option for PTSD. Although this workbook focuses on CBT tools for treating PTSD, it's also important to discuss medication. Please note that the information in this section is not based on clinical expertise but on evidence from published research. This information is for educational purposes and not for self-diagnosing the best medication regimen in trauma symptom reduction.

This workbook cannot review all the various medications available to treat PTSD; however, there is a consensus on the best type of medication in the treatment of PTSD.

A specific group of antidepressant drugs referred to as selective serotonin-reuptake inhibitors (SSRIs) are the first-choice treatment for PTSD because they have proven to be effective. Of the many SSRIs on the market, sertraline and paroxetine both have received approval from the Food and Drug Administration (FDA) to be used in the treatment of PTSD. These drugs tend to specifically decrease reexperiencing, avoidance, and hyperarousal symptoms.

Sertraline (Zoloft): Numerous studies have proven sertraline's effectiveness in reducing PTSD-related symptoms. Studies have shown that this drug can reduce symptoms in as few as 12 weeks.

Paroxetine (Paxil): Research shows paroxetine is effective in treating chronic PTSD and is most powerful when combined with behavioral treatment. In a 2012 study in the *American Journal of Psychiatry*, study participants experienced a greater reduction of their PTSD symptoms when treated with both PE therapy and paroxetine.

Several generic drugs chemically similar to FDA-approved drugs have been shown to be effective in treating PTSD. The following have shown promising effects in reducing PTSD symptoms:

Fluoxetine (Prozac): This antidepressant has been recommended as the first-line "off-label" treatment. In a 2002 study published in the *British Journal of Psychiatry*, researchers found that fluoxetine was helpful in preventing a relapse of PTSD symptoms. More research is required, however, because the results have been inconsistent for reducing PTSD symptoms in individuals.

»

Prazosin (Minipress): Studies have shown that prazosin targets the startle and fear response and can reduce the frequency of trauma-related nightmares. There is limited research on its effect in treating other PTSD symptoms.

Venlafaxine (Effexor): This drug can target multiple symptoms of PTSD. In a 2008 study published in the *International Journal of Neuropsychopharmacology*, participants who took venlafaxine for two weeks saw a decrease in irritability, and those who took it for four weeks saw a reduction in intrusive thoughts. More research is required on venlafaxine, because other studies have shown inconsistent findings.

Rediscover Your Purpose

The goal of this activity is to guide you through your current PTSD journey and recognize that you do not have to continue down the same path you've been using since developing PTSD.

1.   Think of the path that you have been walking on since you had PTSD. What are some of the things you continue to see on this pathway (e.g., poor relationships, always arguing, wanting control)?

----

2.   On this old path, what are some things that prevented you from taking a different direction (e.g., being scared of change, feeling uncomfortable, not knowing how to change)?

----

3. What do you dislike about this path that you have been walking on for a long time (e.g., not being able to enjoy life)?

4. What would you have to do to take a different direction on a different path (e.g., ask for help, experience my suffering)?

5. What are some unforeseen circumstances you may face on this new path (e.g., confronting my thoughts, emotions, and stressors)?

6. What are some unforeseen circumstances you have already conquered (e.g., I survived my trauma)?

   _____

   _____

   _____

   _____

   _____

7. What do you want this new path to look like (e.g., forgiving myself
   for what happened, having one healthy relationship)?

   _____

   _____

   _____

   _____

   _____

8. Where is the final destination of your new path (e.g., being in control
   of my PTSD; experiencing personal growth)?

   _____

   _____

   _____

   _____

   _____

Chapter 10 Takeaways

Life in general is not meant to be easy. Trauma recovery is a lifelong healing process. It is personal and unique to you. To recap, here are the main points:

- Your healing and recovery are a journey.

- You are in control of your PTSD journey.

- Medication has also been helpful in trauma symptom reduction.

- Two antidepressant drugs, sertraline and paroxetine, are the only two FDA-approved drugs for the treatment of PTSD.

- There is an exercise you can do to rediscover your purpose in relation to your trauma and PTSD.

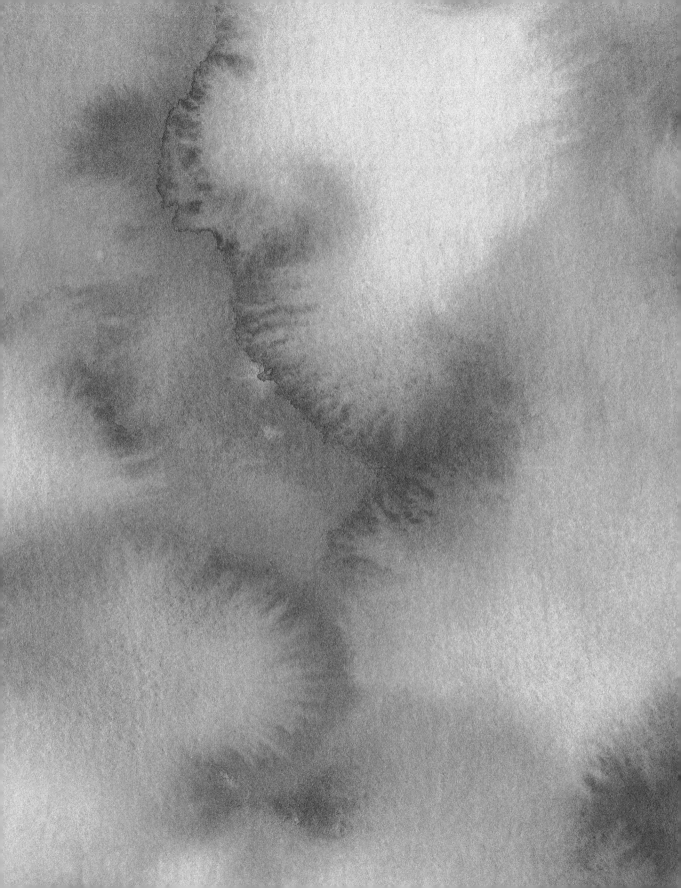

Chapter 11

Your Biggest Challenges

Can you think of all the things that remind you of your trauma? These trauma triggers most likely present themselves in many ways, including in your environment, in conversations, and perhaps in specific places. In this chapter, you will:

- become familiar with trauma triggers,

- understand how trauma triggers affect your brain,

- recognize the difference between internal and external triggers,

- reflect on your own trauma triggers,

- read six different scenarios of PTSD cases and strategies that can be used to overcome trauma triggers, and

- learn additional exercises to use when you are faced with a trauma trigger.

Ready? Let's go.

Overcoming Triggers

After exposure to trauma, the brain easily reads normal life circumstances as dangerous, which can often feel like your brain never shuts down. This is because the brain is continuously scanning the environment for any reminders of the traumatic event that could be perceived as threatening. These trauma reminders are also referred to as trauma triggers.

Trauma triggers feel so powerful because they rely on all our senses. Trauma-related triggers fall into two categories:

Internal: Triggers you feel or experience inside the body. Examples include memories of the traumatic event, intrusive thoughts, emotions, and bodily sensations.

External: Triggers that are reminders outside your body of situations, places, or people related to your traumatic event. Examples include the specific location of the trauma, certain smells, physical features of a person, someone standing behind you, or an argument.

It's important to note that trauma triggers are misperceived threats directly related to the trauma; these trauma triggers are usually things that are objectively safe and don't pose an actual threat to you. For example, a bottle of water is a safe and harmless object. However, if a bottle of water was directly connected to a traumatic event, the brain of the trauma survivor has now labeled a bottle of water as unsafe, harmful, and scary.

The Brain and Trauma Triggers

As you previously learned, there are three specific areas of the brain that are hijacked after a traumatic event (see page 6): the amygdala, hippocampus, and prefrontal cortex. When your brain perceives a trauma trigger, these same areas of the brain are activated.

Amygdala: The amygdala stores the emotions that were experienced during the traumatic event. A trauma trigger reactivates those same emotions.

Hippocampus: The hippocampus stores the memory of the traumatic event. A trauma trigger may reactivate those memories.

Prefrontal cortex: The prefrontal cortex works with the amygdala and reacts by choosing the best course of action to get you away from the perceived danger.

Trauma triggers are always around you, and they can occur with or without your awareness. They can be present at home, work, or even in a social setting. You cannot control when triggers appear. What you can control is how you react to these triggers. It's within your control to view these triggers as factually safe because these trauma triggers are harmless to your life.

Avoiding your trauma triggers may benefit you in the short term. However, avoiding your trauma triggers in the long term can decrease your quality of life.

Internal vs. External Trauma Triggers

Recognizing your trauma triggers can help you become aware of them and challenge them. Use this exercise to help you specify your trauma triggers.

What are your internal trauma triggers?

_____

_____

_____

What are your external trauma triggers?

_____

_____

_____

Easy vs. Difficult Trauma Triggers

Some trauma triggers are less threatening than other trauma triggers.

Which trauma triggers are easier to "deal with," and why?

_____

_____

_____

Which trauma triggers are more challenging to "deal with," and why?

....

....

....

The Impact of Avoiding My Triggers

In this exercise, identify how avoidance of your trauma triggers (e.g., places, people, objects) has impacted your life.

Decisions:

....

....

....

Choices:

....

....

....

Relationships:

....

....

....

Work environment:

....

....

....

View of the world:

_____

_____

_____

Parenting:

_____

_____

_____

School:

_____

_____

_____

Conversations:

_____

_____

_____

Other areas of your life:

_____

_____

_____

Applying CBT Strategies in Real-Life Scenarios

This section of the workbook provides you with an alternative perspective on how to work through your PTSD symptoms. You will read six different scenarios of traumatic events, the PTSD symptoms, and the strategies that the trauma survivor can use to address the trauma trigger and/or PTSD symptom. Remember, trauma triggers can present themselves at any given time and can cause PTSD symptoms to resurface, so being aware of strategies you can use is helpful.

Case Study: Alina, a house fire survivor (nightmares)

When Alina was 12 years old, she was playing with her siblings one day when her mother ran into the room screaming, "We have to get out of the house right now. The house is on fire." Alina dropped her toys, and as she and her family ran out of the house, she saw the kitchen in flames. Outside, Alina watched firefighters and police officers battle the fire. Thankfully, no one was injured, but the fire completely destroyed their house. For the next few months, Alina and her family experienced unstable housing. They lived in shelters and hotels, and stayed with family members.

After the fire, Alina developed symptoms of PTSD. She was scared to sleep alone because she had nightmares about the house fire. Every time Alina heard a fire alarm or police siren, she questioned if there was a house fire. Her mind was preoccupied with the memory as she started to express her intrusive thoughts by drawing pictures with themes related to fire. Alina was able to process her trauma through therapy and her symptoms decreased.

One night years later, Alina's boyfriend, Carlos, was cooking them dinner at his apartment. Alina was having fun and was in a good mood. Suddenly, Carlos stepped away from the stove and the pan quickly caught on fire. Carlos was able to stop the fire from spreading using the nearby fire extinguisher. The pan was destroyed but the fire was stopped.

Alina was unable to sleep because she wanted to avoid having nightmares.

Alina immediately became more alert and her heart started to pound really fast. She asked Carlos to use the fire extinguisher again and make sure the fire was out. She checked to make sure the fire had not spread. That night at her own place, Alina had a nightmare about her apartment catching on fire. She woke up in a sweat and immediately checked her place for fire. The next night she had a nightmare about her boyfriend's apartment catching on fire. For the next few days, Alina struggled to go to sleep because she was scared of having another nightmare.

Alina's unexpected trauma trigger (the pan catching on fire) was misperceived as a threat and caused her to develop nightmares again. Although the nightmares were not about her own trauma, the content of her nightmares was related to her traumatic experience. Alina's nightmares brought back the emotions and memory of the house fire from her childhood, so she was unable to sleep because she wanted to avoid having nightmares.

Mindfulness Checking

Immediately after waking from the nightmare, Alina could have used her five senses to bring her back to the present moment and help her recognize that it was a nightmare. Using four of her five senses to be present in the moment, Alina could have done the following:

Sight: It's dark in my house. I do not see any smoke. I do not see any fire.

Sound: I do not hear anything. It is silent in my home. The smoke alarm is not going off.

Touch: My house is currently cold. I'm holding my blanket, which means that I am presently in my bedroom, not in my kitchen.

Smell: I do not smell any fire.

Label Your Nightmare

Instead of trying to avoid her nightmare, Alina could have tried labeling it, which would have helped her sleep better and directly confront her PTSD symptoms. Alina could have labeled her nightmare in the following ways:

I am currently feeling anxious because I had a nightmare.

My body is sweating because I had a nightmare.

I am safe in the present moment; I had a nightmare.

My nightmare is a reminder that I had a traumatic event happen in the past.

Regain Control after a Nightmare

Posttraumatic nightmares are more intense than regular dreams because these nightmares usually involve details or content from the traumatic event. The goal of this exercise is to help your body return to a calm state so you can have a good night's sleep. While reflecting on your own nightmares, respond to the following questions.

What are some recurrent themes of your nightmares?

How might you use your five senses to engage in mindfulness checking after a nightmare?

Vision:

Touch:

Smell:

Taste:

Hearing:

When you wake up from your nightmare, what are five labels you can give your nightmares?

Case Study: Hugo, sexual abuse survivor (intrusive thoughts)

When Hugo was 11 years old he was sexually abused by a male neighbor during a Thanksgiving family get-together at his parents' house. Hugo never told anyone due to feelings of shame, embarrassment, and self-blame. He started to suspect every adult around him and didn't trust anyone, and also began acting out in school. Over time, Hugo learned to suppress his PTSD symptoms. Although he occasionally experienced PTSD symptoms, he quickly shut them down because he never directly confronted his PTSD.

Years later, Hugo and his girlfriend hosted a family get-together at their house. Hugo's mother brought over homemade pastry. As she placed it on the table, Hugo asked his mother why she had decided to bake. Hugo's mother reminded him the dish was one of his favorite childhood pastries. Over dinner, Hugo's demeanor changed. He became irritable and stopped interacting with the family. Eventually, Hugo disengaged from family conversation and sat in front of the television, unable to concentrate.

> *Hugo had a hard time regaining control of his PTSD because he felt he was reliving his trauma.*

For the next couple of days, Hugo was not himself. He was moody but unable to explain why. Hugo tried everything he could to suppress the intrusive thoughts. He started going to the bar on the way home. One drink turned into two, and eventually, he was spending more time at the bar as he learned that drinking helped him escape the painful memories and thoughts. As the days passed, Hugo's drinking increased, and other areas of his life became impacted. His drinking led to relationship problems with his family and his girlfriend.

Hugo's trauma trigger (smell) reminded him of the sexual abuse and brought back painful images of that day. His quick change in mood occurred because the trigger brought him back to feelings of self-blame, shame, and embarrassment. Hugo had a hard time regaining control of his PTSD because he felt he was reliving his trauma. His only way to escape from these memories was to self-medicate with alcohol, which resulted in additional negative consequences.

Talk to Your Thought or Memory

Rather than finding ways to avoid his intrusive thoughts, Hugo could have confronted them by talking to them. Remember that when you are experiencing an intrusive thought, your brain "tricks" you into thinking that the trauma is happening again. By talking to his thoughts, Hugo could confront thoughts as just thoughts, helping him recognize that the trauma happened in the past and his thoughts were just thoughts. Hugo could have said to himself,

I welcome you every time, thought.

I'm okay with you visiting me right now.

You are just a thought.

Schedule Time for Your Thoughts

Confronting your trauma trigger will help you recognize that you do not have to be afraid of your intrusive thoughts or the trauma-related memory. Scheduling a time to deliberately think about your thought or memory will gradually decrease the anxiety and fear of the thought or memory. Instead of turning to alcohol to avoid his intrusive thoughts, it may have helped Hugo to set aside 10 minutes to just experience the thoughts without judgment. At the end of the 10 minutes, Hugo could learn to let go of those thoughts.

Regain Control of Intrusive Thoughts

You do not have to give your intrusive thoughts power. Giving them power allows the thoughts to dominate and control your life. The more you try to actively stop a thought, the more powerful the thought becomes. By allowing yourself to talk to your thought, you are confronting the thought, acknowledging that it exists, and regaining control. Talking to your thought opens up the opportunity for kindness with yourself.

Here are some ways you can talk to your thoughts:

I welcome you every time, thought.

You can visit as long as you want.

I do not fear you and I will not listen to you.

It is okay that you are here today.

I recognize that you are only a thought.

What are some other ways you can talk to your intrusive thoughts?

_____

_____

_____

You can also schedule a time of the day to just focus on your intrusive thoughts. Allow yourself 10 minutes to have these intrusive thoughts without judgment. Let them enter, and continue to look for more and more of them. If you run out of intrusive thoughts, go back and repeat the ones you've already had.

What is the best time for you to sit down and welcome your intrusive thoughts? Why would this be the best time?

_____

_____

_____

Case Study: Lee, robbed at gunpoint (reexperiencing, flashback)

Lee was walking to his car after work one day when he was approached from behind and robbed at gunpoint. The unidentified man "belittled" him and threatened to kill Lee if he did not give him all his money. Lee quickly reached into his pockets and gave him his wallet. The unidentified man walked away without harming Lee; however, Lee was in such shock that he couldn't find the keys to his car, which were in his pocket. When he got into his car he called 911. He filed a report, but was unable to provide a description of the robber.

Lee had a difficult time not thinking about the event. He made mistakes at work because his brain was preoccupied with the traumatic event. He couldn't sleep at night because he feared for his life. He became alert and on guard, frequently checking his surroundings. Lee even changed his parking spot at work. A few weeks after the incident, his PTSD symptoms subsided.

Lee became more alert and on guard, and started checking his surroundings.

Three months after the traumatic event, Lee had a meeting with his boss and felt "belittled" by him. Lee left the meeting angry and returned to his desk. He avoided seeing his boss for the rest of the day. He was unable to concentrate because his mind was preoccupied with thoughts and memories of the robbery. He felt like he was reliving his trauma because the memory played over and over in his head. As he walked to his car, his trauma memory reminded him that he could potentially get robbed again. He became more alert and on guard, and started checking his surroundings. He held his phone in his hand so that if he was robbed, he could immediately dial 911.

The next day Lee was late to work and was irritable with his coworkers. As he was working on a task, a coworker approached him from behind, which triggered the trauma memory for Lee. His heart started to beat faster and his blood pressure rose, causing him to physically push his coworker away. Due to the behavior, Lee was fired from his job.

Use Power Language

Instead of letting the PTSD take control, Lee could have used power words to help him work through his PTSD. The words we choose to describe our fears, struggles, and ourselves can become powerful tools. Most likely, Lee said to himself, "I can't control my PTSD," which caused him to feel hopeless and his symptoms to worsen. Instead, if he had said, "I can control my PTSD and I'm learning to conquer it," this may have felt empowering and given him a sense of hope, which may have led to a different reaction.

Victim vs. Survivor

Often, trauma survivors refer to themselves as "victims." Lee's intrusive memory may have led him to continue feeling victimized and helpless. If Lee had referred to himself as a "survivor," the memory would have had less power and eventually would have subsided. Referring to himself as a survivor would have felt more empowering than referring to himself as a victim. Using the term "victim" diminishes strength and resiliency, whereas using the term "survivor" conveys that an individual has control and thrives in their environment. Referring to himself as a survivor would have changed the way Lee reacted to his boss and his coworker.

Giving Myself Back the Power

Using power language when your PTSD symptoms revisit can help you regain control and manage your PTSD. These are some examples of power language.

NEGATIVE POWER LANGUAGE	POSITIVE POWER LANGUAGE
I am a victim.	I am a survivor.
I have PTSD.	I have PTSD, but it is treatable.
I can't control PTSD.	I am learning to conquer PTSD.
Nobody understands what I've been through.	Everybody faces their own battles.

What power language are you going to use when your PTSD symptoms revisit?

....

....

....

When you refer to yourself as a victim, what thoughts, feelings, and reactions do you notice in yourself?

....

....

....

When you refer to yourself as a survivor, what thoughts, feelings, and reactions do you notice in yourself?

....

....

....

Case Study: Priya, car accident survivor (avoidance)

Priya was in a car crash four years ago. She was driving her car when she was hit by an SUV, causing her to lose control, and her car to flip over. She was unable to get herself out and had to wait for police and firefighters to rescue her from the car. She suffered a broken leg, but there were no other significant medical complications from the crash.

Immediately after the crash, Priya developed symptoms of PTSD, including intrusive thoughts and nightmares. She refused to drive, and when she got into a vehicle she felt hot and sweaty, and her heart rate increased. She decided not to repair the car, and instead sold it. She avoided everything that reminded her of the crash, including the location. She returned to work a few weeks later but took public transportation. Over time, Priya sought treatment. She developed tools to use when she was faced with a trauma trigger and felt she had her PTSD under control. She eventually purchased a car and got back on the road.

A year later, Priya changed jobs, requiring her to pass by the scene of the crash on her commute. The first day, she passed by the location and felt fine. However, that night she experienced unexplainable restlessness. The next day, she felt really tense on her commute to work, and drove quickly past the scene of the crash. On her way home, Priya had a panic attack in the car.

Priya started taking alternative routes, causing her to arrive late.

Priya began remembering her car crash and reexperiencing the same emotions she felt after the crash. She started taking alternative routes, causing her to arrive late to work. Then, her husband began taking her to work and a coworker would drive her home. Priya started to find excuses to call out from work so she didn't have to get into the car.

Priya realized her trauma trigger was impacting her life. Using what she had learned in therapy, she recognized her trauma trigger was a misperceived fear and she confronted her problem. Eventually, she was able to get behind the wheel again and drive to work. Although she still experiences some physical symptoms as she drives by the crash site, she recognizes that her trigger is a misperceived fear.

Confront Trauma-Related Fears

Actively avoiding trauma triggers may temporarily help alleviate your PTSD symptoms, but it doesn't allow you to work through the problem. You are pushing yourself away from the problem rather than resolving it. Priya could have used the CONFRONT acronym:

Challenge your avoidance

Optimistic perspective of your trauma trigger

Navigate your way through the avoidance

Face the misperceived fear

Remind yourself that the trauma is in the past

Observe your reaction

Name your fear

Tell yourself that you overcame past trauma triggers

Label the Fear

Remember that after traumatic events, the brain scans for any trauma triggers, misperceiving them as fears. Priya recognized her trauma triggers were misperceived fears and that her life was not in actual danger. Priya could have also viewed this objectively by asking herself how someone else would react in this situation.

1. Is my trauma trigger an actual threat?

2. Is my trauma currently happening to me?

3. Is my life currently in danger?

4. If someone next to me were experiencing this trauma trigger, would they react the same way?

Meet Your Trauma Triggers Head-On

When you are engaging in avoidance strategies, you are not directly confronting the fear that the trauma trigger elicits. Use the CONFRONT acronym to help you confront future trauma triggers.

1.   Challenge: How might you **C**hallenge your fears?

_____

_____

_____

2.   Optimistic: In what ways can you be **O**ptimistic about your trauma trigger?

_____

_____

_____

3.   Navigate: In what ways can you **N**avigate yourself through your trauma trigger?

_____

_____

_____

4.   Face: In what way can you **F**ace the misperceived fear?

_____

_____

_____

5.   Remind: What are some ways you can **R**emind yourself that the trauma is in the past?

_____

_____

_____

6. Observe: When you step away and **O**bserve your reaction to the trauma trigger, what can you conclude?

_____

_____

_____

7. Name: What are phrases you can use to **N**ame the fear?

_____

_____

_____

8. Tell: What can you **T**ell yourself about how you have overcome your past trauma triggers?

_____

_____

_____

Label your fears

1. What is one way you can assess if you are in actual danger in your current situation?

_____

_____

_____

2.   What is one way you can assess if you are in misperceived danger in your current situation?

_____

_____

_____

3.   If someone next to you were experiencing this trauma trigger, would they react the same way?

_____

_____

_____

Case Study: Anton, witnessed a shooting (hypervigilance)

Anton and his friends were playing their weekly basketball game at the local park one night when they heard loud bangs. They turned to see a woman running from a man and shouting, "Don't do it! Don't do it!" The man pointed a gun at her and fatally shot her. The man turned, saw Anton and his friends, ran to a waiting car, and drove away. Anton and his friends called 911 and reported what they had witnessed.

Over the next few days, Anton was preoccupied with what he had witnessed. He couldn't fall asleep. He lost interest in playing basketball. He avoided the park. Any time he heard a loud noise, he was easily startled. When he was in a room, he paid careful attention to the exits. Anton turned to his support system to help him cope with the traumatic event. Although his PTSD was still present, he learned how to cope with it.

Any time Anton heard a loud noise, he was easily startled.

Months later, Anton was at the movies with his girlfriend when a character in the film said, "Don't do it! Don't do it!" Anton became uncomfortable and distracted for the rest of the film. On the drive back home, they heard fireworks and Anton became startled. He became hyperaware of his surroundings, fearing that someone was trying to shoot at the car.

That night, Anton eventually fell asleep but was startled awake by his roommate slamming the door. He jumped out of bed with his heart beating. His trauma trigger of that specific phrase from the movie had brought back the memory of the shooting and caused him to become easily startled and hypervigilant.

Scan for Positive Cues

Feeling constantly alert or on guard requires a lot of energy from the body and brain. Instead of focusing your attention on what may be dangerous or unsafe, you could focus your attention on any positive cues in your environment. When Anton was sitting in the movie theater, he could have scanned for positive environmental cues, including the fact that everyone was laughing at the movie and everyone was still in their seats. He also could have asked his girlfriend to confirm that the present moment was safe.

Recognize Your Hypervigilant Responses

Anton formed habits in response to a traumatic event, so that if his life was in danger, he could escape easily. These habits included paying attention to the location of exits, not sitting with his back to the door, staying away from crowds, and being aware of loud noises. If Anton had recognized his habits were a response to a traumatic event, he could have confronted them and worked on changing them. The more you confront your hypervigilant habits, the more your brain will learn that everything is okay and that it doesn't always have to be alert and on guard.

Regain Control of Your Hypervigilance

Think about a time when you experienced hypervigilance. How did you react?

_____

_____

_____

Now reflect on what you wrote and how you might have reacted if you scanned your environment for positive cues at that time?

_____

_____

_____

What are some positive cues that you can remind yourself to look for in your environment?

_____

_____

_____

Hypervigilant habits develop as a way to feel less threatened. Examples of some of these habits include constantly checking to see who is behind you, locking the doors and windows every time you get in your car, not sitting with your back to the door, and scanning people in public for odd or threatening behaviors.

What are your hypervigilant habits?

_____

_____

_____

Which hypervigilant habits are you willing to let go of?

_____

_____

_____

Case Study: Nia, suffered a pregnancy loss (destructive behavior)

Nia and her boyfriend were excited to find out she was pregnant. After the first two trimesters went by easily, they began talking about baby names and picking out furniture for the nursery. Shortly after her week 37 checkup, Nia experienced cramping and bleeding. She and her boyfriend rushed to the hospital, where she learned her pregnancy was no longer viable. After a day in the hospital, she and her boyfriend returned home with empty hands, to a silent and empty nursery room.

Nia was devastated. For months, she avoided driving past hospitals and going to baby showers, and she was angry at every pregnant woman. She even began to have dreams about being pregnant and losing the baby. The memory of the trauma constantly replayed in her mind. She was too ashamed, disappointed, and embarrassed to return to work, so she quit her job.

Nia "numbed" her pain with overeating and self-harming.

Nia felt guilty and blamed herself for the death of the baby. The memories and emotions became so painful that Nia "numbed" her pain with overeating and self-harming. Eventually, Nia sought treatment. Although she continues to struggle with PTSD, she is doing much better. She was prescribed medication, returned to work, and is doing her best every day.

Six months later, Nia learned that a friend was pregnant. She began to cry. The same day, she began having flashbacks of the day she lost her baby. She stopped attending a support group she had joined and returned to unhealthy coping mechanisms and self-harm. The memories were too painful, and she just wanted to escape the memories and emotions.

Use a Support System

Instead of turning to destructive behavior and self-harm, Nia could have used healthy coping strategies, such as finding support from others, to help her overcome the negative effects of her trauma. Using a support network could have helped Nia work through the stressful situation and provided emotional validation.

Support systems can include romantic partners, family members, emergency hotline numbers, therapy, and support groups. Nia had multiple support systems available, including her support group and her boyfriend. However, Nia's trauma trigger became so powerful that she was unable to effectively use this coping mechanism.

Every support network can offer help with your healing and recovery. For example, a therapist can teach you how to use healthy and effective coping strategies. Romantic partners or family members can be there to support you physically and emotionally. If you don't have anyone to turn to, try an emergency hotline number to find treatment providers. These calls are also private and confidential.

Journaling to Replace Maladaptive Behaviors

Expressive writing can help you cope with traumatic events by allowing you to let go of your deepest memories and emotions. It can also help bring attention to the thinking pattern and emotional expression you experience while you are struggling with PTSD. If Nia had turned to a more appropriate behavior, such as journaling, she could have experienced posttraumatic growth. Reflecting on her thoughts and emotions around the trauma could have helped her deal with the pain and grow in positive ways. Journaling is also effective when you share your writing with your therapist. The therapist can help you work through your thought process and emotions.

Find Your Support Network

Having someone to confide in at your most stressful time is important to your well-being. Support networks can help you work through stressful situations and can validate your feelings.

Who is one person and/or group you can talk to about the following?:

- Your trauma: _____

- Your PTSD: _____

- Your trauma-related emotions: ....

- Your trauma triggers: ....

- Helping you work through your PTSD or triggers: ....

- Helping you recognize when you may be having a PTSD symptom: ....

Journaling: If you plan to journal to cope with your PTSD, here are some things you can do to reflect on what you wrote.

1. Put away the expressive writing and set a reminder on your phone to read it one month from the day you set the reminder. When the day arrives, read what you wrote and make edits.

2. After you express yourself, you can shred or burn the journal entry.

3. Ask someone else to read it and have them reflect on the writing with you.

4. Put your expressive writing in an envelope, seal it, stamp it, and ask someone you trust to mail you the letter one month from the day you give it to them.

Chapter 11 Takeaways

Trauma triggers are always going to be around you. Learning how to recognize and overcome them will help you conquer your PTSD. To recap, these are the main points:

- Trauma triggers fall into two categories: internal trauma triggers and external trauma triggers.

- Trauma triggers activate the three brain areas that are well known to PTSD: the amygdala, hippocampus, and prefrontal cortex.

- Trauma triggers can cause various different PTSD reactions.

- There are reflective exercises you can engage in to help you better recognize and safely confront your trauma triggers.

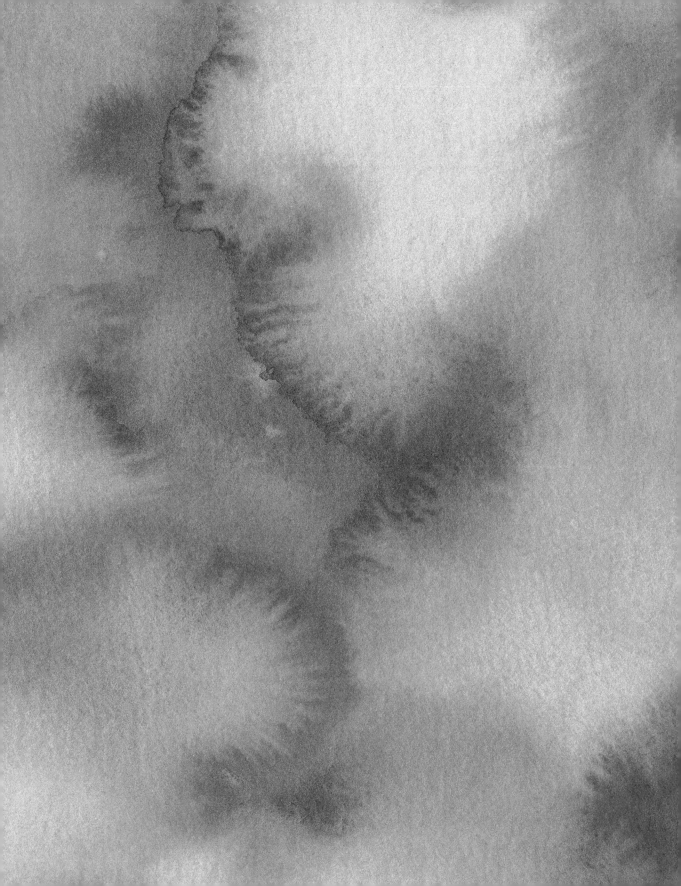

Chapter 12

The Road to Freeing Yourself

Have you ever wondered how some trauma survivors are able to move forward and thrive? Trauma does not have to be a wholly destructive force in a person's life. The ability to thrive after a traumatic event is a result of posttraumatic growth. In this chapter, you will:

- define resiliency and posttraumatic growth,
- become familiar with the five features of posttraumatic growth, and
- engage in exercises that help you recognize your own growth and resiliency.

   Ready? Let's go.

Resilience and Growth

Your ability to remain strong after your traumatic experience is referred to as *resilience*. In its simplest form, resilience is the ability to adapt to negative life experiences and continue with life.

According to research from psychologist Suzanne Kobasa, there are three essential elements to building resilience, and these are referred to as the *three Cs*, or *hardiness*.

1. **Challenge:** Resilient people view their setbacks and/or trauma experiences as challenges rather than paralyzing events, which encourages them to become a better person for having experienced traumatic events. For example, a trauma survivor may reframe their threats as opportunities or view their recovery as a challenge rather than a painful experience.

2. **Commitment:** Resilient people have a sense of purpose and meaning in life and commit to a course of action or "sticking it out" in difficult situations. They view the world as an interesting place and seek involvement in the world. This commitment allows them to keep going. For example, a trauma survivor on the road to recovery may refuse substances due to their commitment to change.

3. **Personal control:** Resilient people strive to gain control of what they can by going into action. Resilient people prioritize situations and events that they do have control over and do not allow things that are out of their control to hijack their thoughts, feelings, and behaviors. Trauma survivors deliberately develop positive attitudes and an optimistic outlook on life. For example, a trauma survivor accepts challenges and may learn that they can have a positive influence over difficult situations and seek alternatives to problems.

Posttraumatic Growth

Some trauma survivors can experience positive psychological change after traumatic life events. This is referred to as posttraumatic growth. This doesn't mean that overcoming your traumatic experience will allow you to return to your pre-trauma life. It means that you will establish a comfortable, integrated perspective of the world that incorporates the traumatic experience, and you will surpass your pre-trauma level of functioning.

Research has shown that trauma survivors who experience positive improvements in the following specific areas have achieved posttraumatic growth:

- Positive trauma identity (self-view)

- Enhancement of relationships

- Willingness to explore new possibilities

- Increased personal strength or feeling stronger

- Spiritual growth and/or greater engagement with fundamental existential questions

- Better appreciation of life

Factors that can increase the likelihood of experiencing posttraumatic growth include:

- the uniqueness of each individual,

- how the survivor manages stressful situations,

- the survivor's process of self-disclosure and response, and

- how much focus and attention the survivor gives to the traumatic event by repetitively thinking about it. This is also referred to as *deliberate rumination*.

I Am a Warrior

Perhaps you might not recognize it right now, but you are a warrior. You have faced challenges in your life, felt like you lost control of your life, and questioned your purpose. What you haven't yet recognized is that you overcame your biggest challenge, are attempting to regain control of your PTSD, and are committed to change. You are a warrior!

What are some challenges you have overcome?

What are ways you have regained control of your PTSD?

What have you committed to? What are you willing to commit to?

My Setbacks Are My Strengths

As you make progress on your PTSD journey, life will throw obstacles in your way. We all have these setbacks. Think of these obstacles as reminders that you have been through more significant experiences in your life. What happens when you fall? You get right back up. If you learn that you can overcome your setbacks, you end up better than you were before.

I know that I am prepared to face any challenge because:

....

....

....

....

I know that if I have a setback, I can control:

....

....

....

....

My setback will not prevent me from achieving:

....

....

....

....

I'm Still Willing to Grow

Experiencing growth does not mean that you have suffered and are ending that pain. It means finding the purpose of pain and looking beyond the struggle. Every day you will learn something new about yourself, your trauma, and the world.

What are five positive things about yourself that are a result of your trauma?

1. ....

2. ....

3. ....

4. ....

5. ....

In what ways are you willing to change your relationships?

....

....

....

....

What have you appreciated about life since you started your healing journey?

....

....

....

....

Since your traumatic experience, what is something new you learned about . . .

Yourself:

....

....

....

....

Your trauma:

....

....

....

....

The world:

....

....

....

....

Create Rituals and Habits to Heal

Being able to thrive in a fast-paced world requires good self-care, or a healthy relationship with yourself. You need to stop and take the time to remind yourself that you are important, too. It's important to take care of your mind and body, not just when you are sick, but on a daily basis. The more self-care you do, the stronger you will become at conquering obstacles and improving your quality of life. Self-care is a deliberate choice, which means that you are actively engaging in an activity that nourishes and maintains an optimal level of well-being.

Having a healthy relationship with yourself allows you to be more mindful of your PTSD. And when symptoms resurface, you can conquer them in healthy and effective ways.

Good self-care includes:

- healthy diet,

- good sleep practice,

- physical exercise,

- relaxation techniques,

- noticing the positives throughout your day, and

- surrounding yourself with healthy relationships.

You can also create your own self-care habits to help you heal and recover from your traumatic experience. Here are a few exercises you can include in your self-care routines.

Your Healing Ritual

Think of your self-care for PTSD as your healing ritual to separate from your trauma. Your healing ritual should be practiced daily so that you can move toward a better and healthier you every day. It can help you restore balance and harmony in your life.

Remember, there is a difference between a ritual and a routine. A ritual is a meaningful practice, has a sense of purpose, can provide comfort, and empowers you to think more clearly and feel in control of your life. A routine is a task you engage in as part of your day. Your healing ritual can include anything that holds personal significance to you.

Daily Rituals

Think of something you do on a daily basis that can be turned into a daily ritual. What is a daily ritual that you can commit to (e.g., waking up with a smile on my face; going for a morning walk; listening to the same song every day; staying away from my phone for 30 minutes)?

Gratitude

Gratitude is a great self-care activity. Research has shown that practicing daily gratitude is associated with greater happiness. Giving thanks creates positive emotions, good experiences, and can help you deal with adversity.

For each of your five senses, write down one thing for which you are grateful.

I am grateful that I can taste_____

I am grateful that I can hear_____

I am grateful that I can see_____

I am grateful that I can smell_____

I am grateful that I can touch or feel _____

Complaint-Free Day

Complaints can carry destructive power because they influence your thoughts, feelings, and actions. People complain for various reasons, including needing attention, removing responsibility, and putting people down to feel more important. Commit to one complaint-free day. What would that day look like? Try it out!

Your Spiritual Practice

Spirituality can be a source of comfort and support for people who have experienced trauma. It can help them better understand why the trauma happened and can lead to new and transformational goals and priorities. It is possible for those who are not religious or who are actively atheistic to experience spiritual growth, as well. They tend to have a greater engagement with the existence of life.

A spiritual practice is personal, as is any ritual that connects you to the real you. Spiritual self-care is different for everyone. For some, spiritual self-care may be found in the tenets of religion, while for others, spiritual self-care may be found in nature. Either way, engaging in spiritual self-care encourages you to examine yourself on a deeper and more aware level. Research has documented that many people draw on spiritual teachings, beliefs or values, and practices while coping with trauma.

Defining Your Spirituality

What does spiritual self-care mean to you?

When would be the best time for you to engage in spiritual self-care?

How can your spiritual self-care improve your well-being, PTSD, and obstacles you may encounter?

The Sacred Mantra

A mantra is a word, phrase, verse, or prayer that helps train your mind to pay attention and focus on the present moment. Think of your sacred mantra as a source of unconditional support.

What is your sacred mantra that speaks to you and has a personal connection to your inner peace?

_____

_____

_____

_____

_____

Daily Trauma Affirmation

Reflect at the end of the day to prepare yourself for the night. When you are done reflecting on your day, you can conclude that you conquered your trauma by repeating an affirmation. Here is an example of an affirmation:

I cannot change my trauma and the decisions I have made in the past. I am thankful for being a survivor and for being present in the moment of another day. I accept the challenges and successes that came my way. I know I tried the best that I could with what I have and what I know. Tomorrow is a new day to conquer.

What is your daily trauma affirmation?

_____

_____

_____

_____

_____

Your Creative Release

Creative release can be a safe way to express the pain and suffering that you've experienced as a trauma survivor. It has the power to aid in healing and can be expressed in positive ways. Creative expression can occur in many ways, including through music, creative writing, flower arranging, art, and gardening. Remember, being creative doesn't mean you have to produce a sculptural masterpiece or a symphony.

Creative release can build self-confidence, express hidden emotions, allow you to de-stress, and provide an overall sense of control, power, and freedom. Creativity can give trauma survivors a voice to express their trauma-related thoughts, feelings, and memories.

Music Playlist

What songs would you use to describe your traumatic event?

What songs would you use to describe your feelings related to the traumatic event?

What songs would you use to describe your PTSD journey?

Finish the Story Differently

Your trauma memory most likely ends at the point when you felt defeated. However, that does not have to be where the story ends.

How would your story change if your memory focused on how you survived the trauma? Write down a different ending that includes your survival.

Past, Present, and Future PTSD Self-Image

Sometimes we forget our struggles and how much they have shaped us. Use this exercise to reflect on your past, present, and future self-image. Describe your self-image prior to your trauma, your current self-image, and what you want your self-image to look like in the future.

Describe your past self-image.

_____

_____

_____

_____

Describe your present self-image.

_____

_____

_____

_____

Describe your future self-image.

_____

_____

_____

_____

Revisiting Your Symptoms

As you've worked your way through this workbook, you will notice a change in your thinking and perhaps a change in the way you perceive the world. Most importantly, you should feel stronger and better than you did prior to opening this book. By now, you should be able to recognize your PTSD symptoms and how the loss of control over your PTSD has impacted multiple areas of your life.

You have likely now reached a point where you can use the coping tools in your toolbox to regain control so that PTSD is no longer controlling you. If you haven't reached this point yet, it's okay. Give yourself as many chances as you need to go back and try again. Although you can't go back in time, you can always go back to any page in this workbook.

Now that you've worked through the strategies and exercises, let's revisit your symptoms to determine their current severity. Remember, every trauma survivor is going to be impacted differently and display different symptoms. There is no one identical PTSD symptom report. If 10 people with PTSD were lined up and asked to describe their symptoms, everyone's answer would be different.

Symptom decline will occur over time. You have to be patient with yourself. Remember, trauma recovery is a process. You cannot work through all the symptoms at once. Each symptom will vary in frequency, intensity, and severity. The more you practice using your new coping tools, the more likely it is that your symptoms will decline over time.

Exposure to Trauma

1.   Go back to chapter 3 and review your exposure to trauma checklist (see page 23). How many symptoms did you check off for exposure to trauma?

     1   2   3   4   5   6   6+

2.   How much has this trauma been impacting you in the past week?

     Never   Rarely   Sometimes   Often   Always

3.   How much has this trauma been impacting you in the past month?

     Never   Rarely   Sometimes   Often   Always

4.   How much has this trauma been impacting you in the past year?

     Never   Rarely   Sometimes   Often   Always

5.   How much has this trauma impacted other areas of your life?

Never   Rarely   Sometimes   Often   Always

If your responses are more toward the never/rarely side, your trauma has not had a significant impact on you. If your responses are more toward the often/always side, your trauma has impacted you and continues to impact your well-being.

Question 5 reflects other domains of your life, such as work, relationships, school, and so forth. If you responded with never/rarely, your trauma has not impacted these areas. If you responded with often/always, your traumatic experience is impacting not just your psychological well-being but other important areas of your life, as well.

Intrusive Thoughts and Nightmares

In the following checklist, have any of the symptoms listed occurred within the past week?

INTRUSIVE MEMORIES	NEVER	SOMETIMES	ALL THE TIME
Does your trauma randomly pop into your head?			
Do you fear this memory?			
Do you experience physiological responses (increased heart rate, increased blood pressure, sweatiness) when you have an intrusive thought?			
Does the intrusive memory cause distress?			
FLASHBACKS	NEVER	SOMETIMES	ALL THE TIME
Do you feel like you are reliving your trauma when you have a trauma memory?			

	NEVER	SOMETIMES	ALL THE TIME
Does your intrusive memory include vivid and graphic details?			
Do you feel like your trauma memory is a movie replaying in your head?			
DISSOCIATION	**NEVER**	**SOMETIMES**	**ALL THE TIME**
Do you lose touch with reality when you think of your trauma memory?			
Do you "space out" when you have a trauma memory?			
Are you unable to remember anything for a period of time?			
Do you feel disconnected or detached from your emotions?			
NIGHTMARES	**NEVER**	**SOMETIMES**	**ALL THE TIME**
Do you have vivid dreams of your trauma?			
Do you wake up in a sweat?			
Do you wake up in fear?			
Do you avoid going to sleep because you do not want to have dreams of your trauma?			
Do you have dreams related to your trauma content?			
Do you have dreams of being hurt or killed?			

If most of your responses are "never," you may be experiencing mild reexperiencing symptoms. If most of your responses are "sometimes," you may be experiencing moderate reexperiencing symptoms. If most of your responses are "all the time," you may be experiencing severe reexperiencing symptoms.

Avoidance

In the following checklist, have any of the symptoms listed occurred within the past week?

AVOIDANCE OF EMOTIONS	NEVER	SOMETIMES	ALL THE TIME
Do you avoid trauma-related feelings?			
Do you find other ways to cope with your trauma-related feelings?			
Have you ever expressed feeling "numb"?			
AVOIDANCE OF MEMORY	NEVER	SOMETIMES	ALL THE TIME
Do you avoid trauma-related memories?			
Do you find other ways to cope with your trauma-related memories?			
Do you find yourself frequently stating, "I can't remember what happened"?			
AVOIDANCE OF THOUGHTS	NEVER	SOMETIMES	ALL THE TIME
Do you avoid trauma-related thoughts?			
Do you find yourself frequently stating, "I don't think about it"?			
Do you find other ways to cope with your trauma-related thoughts?			
TRIGGERS	NEVER	SOMETIMES	ALL THE TIME
Do you avoid people that remind you of your trauma?			
Do you avoid conversations that remind you of your trauma?			

	NEVER	SOMETIMES	ALL THE TIME
Do you avoid relationships because of your trauma?			
Do you avoid places that remind you of your trauma?			
Do you avoid any objects (i.e., foods, scented products, clothing) that remind you of your trauma?			

If most of your responses are "never," you may be experiencing mild avoidance symptoms. If most of your responses are "sometimes," you may be experiencing moderate avoidance symptoms. If most of your responses are "all the time," you may be experiencing severe avoidance symptoms.

Changes in Mood and Thoughts

In the following checklist, have any of the symptoms listed occurred within the past week?

NEGATIVE SELF-VIEW	NEVER	SOMETIMES	ALL THE TIME
Do you view yourself in a negative way?			
Is it hard to find positive qualities about yourself?			
Do you view yourself as worthless?			
Do you view yourself as less deserving?			
Do you view the world as unsafe?			
Do you criticize yourself?			
Do you have more negative than positive views of yourself?			
Do you have more negative than positive views of the world?			

»

SELF-BLAME	NEVER	SOMETIMES	ALL THE TIME
Do you blame yourself for your trauma?			
NEGATIVE AFFECT	**NEVER**	**SOMETIMES**	**ALL THE TIME**
Do you feel ashamed because of your trauma?			
Do you feel embarrassed because of your trauma?			
Are you frequently in fear?			
Do you feel angry most of the time?			
Is it hard to experience positive feelings?			
DIMINISHED INTEREST IN ACTIVITIES	**NEVER**	**SOMETIMES**	**ALL THE TIME**
Since your trauma, have you lost interest in things?			
Since your trauma, is it hard to find pleasure in anything?			
POOR RELATIONSHIPS	**NEVER**	**SOMETIMES**	**ALL THE TIME**
Since your trauma, is it hard to trust others?			
Since your trauma, do you feel "different" from others?			
Since your trauma, do you feel that nobody can understand you?			
Since your trauma, do you feel like there is no one you can rely on?			
INABILITY TO EXPERIENCE POSITIVE EMOTIONS	**NEVER**	**SOMETIMES**	**ALL THE TIME**
Is it hard to experience positive feelings?			

Do you experience more negative than positive feelings?			
Is it hard to experience joy or happiness?			

If most of your responses are "never," you may be experiencing mild changes in mood and thoughts symptoms. If most of your responses are "sometimes," you may be experiencing moderate changes in mood and thoughts symptoms. If most of your responses are "all the time," you may be experiencing severe changes in mood and thoughts symptoms.

Anger, Arousal, and Reactivity

In the following checklist, have any of the symptoms listed occurred within the past week?

IRRITABILITY AND AGGRESSION	NEVER	SOMETIMES	ALL THE TIME
Do you feel angry all the time?			
Do you use phrases such as "lash out," "short temper," or "blackout"?			
Do you feel irritable all the time?			
RISKY AND SELF-DESTRUCTIVE BEHAVIOR	NEVER	SOMETIMES	ALL THE TIME
Have you ever intentionally cut yourself to escape your trauma?			
Have you intentionally scratched or hit yourself to escape your trauma?			
Have you used drugs or alcohol to avoid your trauma?			
Have you been hypersexual (e.g., sex with multiple partners, unprotected sex)?			

»

Have you restricted your food intake, binged, or purged?			
HYPERVIGILANCE	NEVER	SOMETIMES	ALL THE TIME
Do you frequently pay attention to your surroundings?			
Do you frequently feel "on edge"?			
Do you feel unsafe at all times?			
Is it hard to trust others?			
HEIGHTENED STARTLE RESPONSE	NEVER	SOMETIMES	ALL THE TIME
Do you become easily startled?			
Do you become easily jumpy?			
DIFFICULTY CONCENTRATING	NEVER	SOMETIMES	ALL THE TIME
Is it hard to focus because of your trauma?			
Do your intrusive memories prevent you from staying focused?			
Is it hard to maintain conversations because you are thinking about your trauma?			
Can you perform simple tasks without losing focus because you are thinking of your trauma?			
DIFFICULTY WITH SLEEP	NEVER	SOMETIMES	ALL THE TIME
Have you ever tried to avoid sleep in order to not experience nightmares?			
Do you fear going to sleep because of your trauma?			

If most of your responses are "never," you may be experiencing mild arousal and reactivity symptoms. If most of your responses are "sometimes," you may be experiencing moderate arousal and reactivity symptoms. If most of your responses are "all the time," you may be experiencing severe arousal and reactivity symptoms.

Anxiety, Depression, and Panic Attacks

This exercise is meant to give you a baseline of possible symptoms in addition to PTSD. Please note that these questions are not to self-diagnose anxiety, depression, or substance abuse. Your mental health provider can accurately make that diagnosis. This exercise is meant to help you recognize if your anxiety, depression, and substance abuse are directly related to your trauma or if these symptoms are independent of PTSD.

ANXIETY	YES	IF YES, IS THE SYMPTOM TRAUMA RELATED?	NO
Do you worry excessively?			
Do you feel restless?			
Do you have concentration impairment?			
Do you experience physical symptoms?			
Is there an identified stressor when you worry?			
Does your worry cause you sleep impairment?			
Is it hard to control your worry?			
DEPRESSION	YES	IF YES, IS THE SYMPTOM TRAUMA RELATED?	NO
Do you have a depressed mood most of the day?			
Do you feel sad?			
Do you feel hopeless?			

»

	YES	IF YES, IS THE SYMPTOM TRAUMA RELATED?	NO
Do you feel irritable?			
Do you have thoughts of self-harm?			
Have you lost interest or pleasure in activities?			
Have you had a change in appetite?			
Have you had a change in sleep?			
Have you felt inappropriate guilt?			
Have you had suicidal thoughts?			
Have you felt loss of energy or fatigue?			
Have you experienced slowed-down thoughts or a reduction in physical movement?			
SUBSTANCE ABUSE	**YES**	**IF YES, IS THE SYMPTOM TRAUMA RELATED?**	**NO**
Do you have cravings to use drugs/alcohol?			
Do you want to cut down or stop but have difficulty trying to cut down or stop?			
Do you take drugs/alcohol in larger amounts or for longer periods of time?			
Has drugs/alcohol impaired other areas of your life?			
Do you continue to use drugs/alcohol even if it causes problems in relationships?			

Do you use drugs/alcohol even when it puts you in danger?			
Do you continue to use drugs/alcohol even if you have a physical or psychological condition?			
Do you experience withdrawal symptoms?			

If most of your responses to the questions related to anxiety, depression, and substance abuse are "yes" and "trauma related," the anxiety and depression are manifesting as a result of your traumatic experience. If you answered "yes" but did not indicate "trauma related," you may be struggling with a diagnosis in addition to PTSD.

Thriving with PTSD

Everyone at some point in their life will experience a traumatic event. A majority of these individuals will recover from this traumatic event with no disruption in other areas of life. However, some trauma survivors go on to develop symptoms of PTSD. Over time, untreated PTSD almost always impacts an individual's quality of life.

You may not be ready to face your PTSD in therapy, but by picking up this book, you are ready to face your PTSD individually. That's empowering. Using this workbook as a self-help guide to treat your PTSD, you have demonstrated that you, not the PTSD, have the power and control to make choices. You have been given multiple tools for your CBT toolbox and have access to them at all times. By getting this far in the book, you have demonstrated that you are ready to be in control of your PTSD.

Think back to the first time you used a CBT tool and how good you felt afterward. You felt like you finally got a hold of the PTSD. It felt like the first time you beat that dark cloud that has been hovering over you since the traumatic event. Imagine how amazing you will feel the more experienced you become at using your tools. If you forget your tools, you can refer back to this workbook at any point in time.

I want to emphasize again that it takes time to regain control of your PTSD. Your trauma journey wasn't an easy one, but your road to healing and recovery will be an empowering one. For the longest time you have been traveling down the same path over and over again. It is time to take a different path. This new path will allow you to experience a positive transformation following your trauma, also referred to as posttraumatic growth. On this new path, you will no longer feel a constant need to "survive"; instead, you will actually thrive.

If you have finished working through this workbook and have not experienced any change in symptom reduction, or perhaps have experienced only minimal change in symptom reduction, that is okay. You can always return to this workbook and try again. Or perhaps it is time to allow a mental health professional to join you, and guide you on your PTSD journey.

Resources

In addition to this workbook, there are resources that can help you learn more about trauma, PTSD, and mental health. I have found the following resources to be helpful for those struggling with PTSD.

Find a Trauma Therapist

Finding the right fit with a therapist can feel difficult. The best way to find a trauma therapist is through PsychologyToday.com.

When looking for a trauma therapist, here are a few things to consider:

- Do they specialize in trauma-related therapy?

- Do they have CBT certifications?

- Does their profile or website focus on healing trauma survivors?

Getting help is not a sign of weakness or vulnerability. It is a sign that you are ready to own your PTSD and control it. Therapy is confidential and is a safe place to process this daunting memory. If therapy is the only safe place that allows you to heal from trauma, let it be the only place.

PsychologyToday.com is also a great place to find reading material related to mental health. The site can also help you find a treatment center, psychiatrist, and even a support group.

If you are looking for virtual therapy, you can refer to these websites:

- BetterHelp.com

- TalkSpace.com

- PrideCounseling.com

You can also contact your insurance provider or access their website to be connected with a therapist.

Podcasts

Podcasts are a great interactive tool that can inspire, provide an opportunity for personal growth, and help you stay educated and informed. Because they are usually a recorded conversation between two or more individuals, they can feel more personal than one person reporting.

Transforming Trauma: This podcast is about thriving after trauma. Although the podcast focuses on complex trauma, it is a podcast that any trauma survivor can relate to.

The Mental Illness Happy Hour: On this podcast, you will hear stories from noted figures and celebrities about their experiences with mental illness or trauma.

Books

Books provide a wealth of knowledge and can be helpful during our most difficult times. You can become more informed about PTSD or feel empowered after reading a trauma survivor's story.

The Body Keeps the Score: Brain, Mind, and Body in the Healing of Trauma by Bessel A. van der Kolk, M.D.

The Deepest Well: Healing the Long-Term Effects of Childhood Adversity by Nadine Burke Harris, M.D.

It Didn't Start with You: How Inherited Family Trauma Shapes Who We Are and How to End the Cycle by Mark Wolynn

TED Talks

TED Talks are interesting and knowledgeable lectures, including topics related to PTSD, trauma, resiliency, and posttraumatic growth.

"How Childhood Trauma Affects Health Across a Lifetime," Dr. Nadine Burke Harris. www.youtube.com/watch?v=95ovlJ3dsNk

"My Philosophy for a Happy Life," Sam Berns. www.youtube.com/watch?v=36m1o-tM05g

"The Surprising Science of Happiness," Dan Gilbert. https://www.youtube.com/watch?v=4q1dgn_C0AU

"What Trauma Taught Me about Resilience," Charles Hunt. https://www.youtube.com/watch?v=3qELiw_1Ddg

Mental Health Apps

There are several apps available that can give you tools, education, and techniques to overcome your challenge.

Calm: This meditation app offers various tools to help you de-stress, including meditation and breathing programs.

Happify: This app is all about playing games designed to help you overcome negative thoughts and stress, and build resiliency.

PTSD Coach: This app offers various resources and allows you to customize tools based on your own needs and preferences.

What's Up?: This app uses CBT and ACT methods to help you cope.

References

Chapter 1

Brooks, Matthew, Nicola Graham-Kevan, Sarita Robinson, and Michelle Lowe. "Trauma Characteristics and Posttraumatic Growth: The Mediating Role of Avoidance Coping, Intrusive Thoughts, and Social Support." *Psychological Trauma: Theory, Research, Practice, and Policy* 11, no. 2 (2019): 232–238. doi.org/10.1037/tra0000372.

Center for Substance Abuse Treatment (US). "Trauma-Informed Care in Behavioral Health Services" in *Treatment Improvement Protocol (TIP) Series*, No. 57. Rockville, MD: Substance Abuse and Mental Health Services Administration (US), 2014. (Available from ncbi.nlm.nih.gov/books/NBK207201)

Dalgleish, Tim, Beatrijs Hauer, and Willem Kuyken. "The Mental Regulation of Autobiographical Recollection in the Aftermath of Trauma." *Current Directions in Psychological Science* 17, no. 4 (2008): 259–263. Accessed July 11, 2020.

Kessler, R. C., S. Aguilar-Gaxiola, J. Alonso, C. Benjet, E. J. Bromet, G. Cardoso, et al. (2017). "Trauma and PTSD in the WHO World Mental Health Surveys." *European Journal of Psychotraumatology*, 8, no. S5 (2017): 1353383. doi.org/10.1080/20008198.2017.1353383.

Kim, E. J., B. Pellman, and J. J. Kim. "Stress Effects on the Hippocampus: A Critical Review." *Learning & Memory* 22, no. 9 (2015): 411–416. doi.org/10.1101/lm.037291.114.

Kolassa, Iris-Tatjana, and Thomas Elbert. "Structural and Functional Neuroplasticity in Relation to Traumatic Stress." *Current Directions in Psychological Science* 16, no. 6 (2007): 321–325. Accessed July 13, 2020. jstor.org/stable/20183228.

Lowe, Sarah R., Peter James, Mariana C. Arcaya, Mira D. Vale, Jean E. Rhodes, Alinat Rich-Edwards, et al. "Do Levels of Posttraumatic Growth Vary by Type of Traumatic Event Experienced? An Analysis of the Nurses' Health Study II." *Psychological Trauma: Theory, Research, Practice, and Policy* (2020). doi.org/10.1037/tra0000554.

Marks, Elizabeth H., Anna R. Franklin, and Lori A. Zoellner. "Can't Get It Out of My Mind: A Systematic Review of Predictors of Intrusive Memories of Distressing Events." *Psychological Bulletin* 144, no. 6 (2018): 584–640. doi.org/10.1037/bul0000132.

Oulton, Jacinta M., Deryn Strange, Reginald D. V. Nixon, and Melanie K. T. Takarangi. "PTSD and the Role of Spontaneous Elaborative 'Nonmemories.'" *Psychology of*

Consciousness: Theory, Research, and Practice 5, no. 4 (2018): 398–413. doi.org/10.1037/cns0000158.

Schultebraucks, Katharina, Felicitas Rombold-Bruehl, Katja Wingenfeld, Julian Hellmann-Regen, Christian Otte, and Stefan Roepke. "Heightened Biological Stress Response during Exposure to a Trauma Film Predicts an Increase in Intrusive Memories." Journal of Abnormal Psychology 128, no. 7 (2019): 645–657. doi.org/10.1037/abn0000440.

Shin, L. M., S. L. Rauch, and R. K. Pitman. "Amygdala, Medial Prefrontal Cortex, and Hippocampal Function in PTSD." Annals of the New York Academy of Sciences 1071, no. 1 (2006): 67–79. doi.org/10.1196/annals.1364.007.

Williams, L. M., A. H. Kemp, K. Felmingham, M. Barton, G. Olivieri, A. Peduto, et al. "Trauma Modulates Amygdala and Medial Prefrontal Responses to Consciously Attended Fear." NeuroImage 29, no. 2 (2006): 347–357. doi.org/10.1016/j.neuroimage.2005.03.047.

Chapter 2

American Psychiatric Association. Diagnostic and Statistical Manual of Mental Disorders, Fifth Edition. Arlington, VA: American Psychiatric Association, 2013.

Bassett, D., D. Buchwald, and S. Manson. "Posttraumatic Stress Disorder and Symptoms among American Indians and Alaska Natives: A Review of the Literature." Social Psychiatry and Psychiatric Epidemiology 49, no. 3 (2014): 417–433. doi.org/10.1007/s00127-013-0759-y.

Blacker, C. J., M. A. Frye, E. Morava, T. Kozicz, and M. Veldic. "A Review of Epigenetics of PTSD in Comorbid Psychiatric Conditions." Genes 10, no. 2 (2019): 140. doi.org/10.3390/genes10020140.

Breslau, Naomi. "The Epidemiology of Trauma, PTSD, and Other Posttrauma Disorders." Trauma, Violence & Abuse 10, no. 3 (2009): 198–210. Accessed July 11, 2020. jstor.org/stable/26636190.

Dorrington, S., H. Zavos, H. Ball, P. McGuffin, A. Sumathipala, S. Siribaddana, et al. "Family Functioning, Trauma Exposure and PTSD: A Cross Sectional Study." Journal of Affective Disorders, 245 (2019): 645–652. doi.org/10.1016/j.jad.2018.11.056.

Horwitz, Allan V. PTSD: A Short History. Baltimore, MD: John Hopkins University Press, 2018.

Javidi, H., and M. Yadollahie. "Post-traumatic Stress Disorder." International Journal of Occupational and Environmental Medicine 3, no. 1 (2012): 2–9.

Kasper, Violet. "Posttraumatic Stress Disorder: Diagnosis, Prevalence, and Research Advances." Sociological Focus 35, no. 1 (2002): 97–108. Accessed July 11, 2020. jstor.org/stable/20832154.

Sibrava, Nicholas J., Andri S. Bjornsson, A. Carlos I. Pérez Benítez, Ethan Moitra, Risa B. Weisberg, and Martin B. Keller. "Posttraumatic Stress Disorder in African American and Latinx Adults: Clinical Course and the Role of Racial and Ethnic Discrimination." *American Psychologist* 74, no. 1 (2019): 101–116. doi.org/10.1037/amp0000339.

Chapter 3

American Psychiatric Association. *Diagnostic and Statistical Manual of Mental Disorders*, Fifth Edition. Arlington, VA: American Psychiatric Association, 2013.

Barbieri, A., F. Visco-Comandini, D. Alunni Fegatelli, C. Schepisi, V. Russo, F. Calò, et al. "Complex Trauma, PTSD and Complex PTSD in African Refugees." *European Journal of Psychotraumatology* 10, no. 1 (2019): 1700621. doi.org/10.1080/20008198.2019.1700621.

Blanchard, Anika Wiltgen, Katrina Rufino, Elizabeth Hartwig Rea, Kieran Paddock, and Michelle A. Patriquin. "Nightmares in Adult Psychiatric Inpatients with and without History of Interpersonal Trauma." *Dreaming* 30, no. 2 (2020): 107–119. doi.org/10.1037/drm0000134.

Boscarino, Joseph A., and Richard E. Adams. "Peritraumatic Panic Attacks and Health Outcomes Two Years after Psychological Trauma: Implications for Intervention and Research." *Psychiatry Research* 167, no. 1–2 (2009): 139–150. doi.org/10.1016/j.psychres.2008.03.019.

Carroll, Kathryn K., Ashton M. Lofgreen, Darian C. Weaver, Philip Held, Brian J. Klassen, Dale L. Smith, et al. "Negative Posttraumatic Cognitions among Military Sexual Trauma Survivors." *Journal of Affective Disorders* 238 (2018): 88–93. doi.org/10.1016/j.jad.2018.05.024.

Carter, Sierra, Abigail Powers, and Bekh Bradley. "PTSD and Self-Rated Health in Urban Traumatized African American Adults: The Mediating Role of Emotion Regulation." *Psychological Trauma: Theory, Research, Practice, and Policy* 12, no. 1 (2020): 84–91. doi.org/10.1037/tra0000472.

Contractor, Ateka A., Nicole H. Weiss, Paula Dranger, Camilo Ruggero, and Cherie Armour. "PTSD's Risky Behavior Criterion: Relation with DSM-5 PTSD Symptom Clusters and Psychopathology." *Psychiatry Research* 252 (2017): 215–222. doi.org/10.1016/j.psychres.2017.03.008.

El-Solh, Ali A. "Management of Nightmares in Patients with Posttraumatic Stress Disorder: Current Perspectives." *Nature and Science of Sleep* 10 (2018): 409–420. doi.org/10.2147/nss.s166089.

Ferrari, Giulia, Gene Feder, Roxane Agnew-Davies, Jayne E. Bailey, Sandra Hollinghurst, Louise Howard, et al. "Psychological Advocacy towards Healing (PATH): A Randomized

Controlled Trial of a Psychological Intervention in a Domestic Violence Service Setting." *PLOS ONE* 13, no. 11 (2018). doi.org/10.1371/journal.pone.0205485.

Fleurkens, Pascal, Mike Rinck, and Agnes van Minnen. "Implicit and Explicit Avoidance in Sexual Trauma Victims Suffering from Posttraumatic Stress Disorder: A Pilot Study." *European Journal of Psychotraumatology* 5, no. 1 (2014): 21359. doi.org/10.3402/ejpt.v5.21359.

Flory, Janine. D., and Rachel Yehuda. "Comorbidity Between Post-Traumatic Stress Disorder and Major Depressive Disorder: Alternative Explanations and Treatment Considerations." *Dialogues in Clinical Neuroscience,* 17, no. 2 (2015): 141–150.

Fox, Robert, Philip Hyland, Joanna McHugh Power, and Andrew N. Coogan. "Patterns of Comorbidity Associated with *ICD-11* PTSD among Older Adults in the United States." *Psychiatry Research* 290 (2020): 113171. doi.org/10.1016/j.psychres.2020.113171.

Giourou, Evangelia, Maria Skokou, Stuart P. Andrew, Konstantina Alexopoulou, Philippos Gourzis, and Eleni Jelastopulu. "Complex Posttraumatic Stress Disorder: The Need to Consolidate a Distinct Clinical Syndrome or to Reevaluate Features of Psychiatric Disorders Following Interpersonal Trauma?" *World Journal of Psychiatry* 8, no. 1 (2018): 12–19. doi.org/10.5498/wjp.v8.i1.12.

Held, Philip, Gina P. Owens, and Scott E. Anderson. "The Interrelationships among Trauma-Related Guilt and Shame, Disengagement Coping, and PTSD in a Sample of Treatment-Seeking Substance Users." *Traumatology* 21, no. 4 (2015): 285–292. doi.org/10.1037/trm0000050.

Hesse, Amy R. "Secondary Trauma: How Working with Trauma Survivors Affects Therapists." *Clinical Social Work Journal* 30 (2002): 293–309.

Horwitz, Adam G., Philip Held, Brian J. Klassen, Niranjan S. Karnik, Mark H. Pollack, and Alyson K. Zalta. "Posttraumatic Cognitions and Suicidal Ideation among Veterans Receiving PTSD Treatment." *Cognitive Therapy and Research* 42, no. 5 (2018): 711–719. doi.org/10.1007/s10608-018-9925-6.

Jones, Alyssa C., Christal L. Badour, C. Alex Brake, Caitlyn O. Hood, and Matthew T. Feldner. "Facets of Emotion Regulation and Posttraumatic Stress: An Indirect Effect via Peritraumatic Dissociation." *Cognitive Therapy and Research* 42, no. 4 (2018): 497–509. doi.org/10.1007/s10608-018-9899-4.

Joscelyne, Amy, Siobhan McLean, Juliette Drobny, and Richard A. Bryant. "Fear of Memories: The Nature of Panic in Posttraumatic Stress Disorder." *European Journal of Psychotraumatology* 3, no. 1 (2012): 19084. doi.org/10.3402/ejpt.v3i0.19084.

Kim-Spoon, Jungmeen, Mary E. Haskett, Gregory S. Longo, and Rachel Nice. "Longitudinal Study of Self-Regulation, Positive Parenting, and Adjustment Problems among Physically Abused Children." *Child Abuse & Neglect* 36, no. 2 (2012): 95–107. doi.org/10.1016/j.chiabu.2011.09.016.

Kolk, Bessel A. van Der. "Developmental Trauma Disorder: Toward a Rational Diagnosis for Children with Complex Trauma Histories." *Psychiatric Annals* 35, no. 5 (2005): 401–408. doi.org/10.3928/00485713-20050501-06.

Kumar, Shaina A., Bethany L. Brand, and Christine A. Courtois. "The Need for Trauma Training: Clinicians' Reactions to Training on Complex Trauma." *Psychological Trauma: Theory, Research, Practice, and Policy* (2019). doi.org/10.1037/tra0000515.

Levin, Andrew P., and Scott Greisberg. "Vicarious Trauma in Attorneys" *Pace Law Review* 24, no. 1 (2003): 245–252. digitalcommons.pace.edu/plr/vol24/iss1/11.

Mantua, Janna, Steven M. Helms, Kris B. Weymann, Vincent F. Capaldi, and Miranda M. Lim. "Sleep Quality and Emotion Regulation Interact to Predict Anxiety in Veterans with PTSD." *Behavioural Neurology* 2018 (2018): 1–10. doi.org/10.1155/2018/7940832.

Marks, Elizabeth H., Anna R. Franklin, and Lori A. Zoellner. "Can't Get It Out of My Mind: A Systematic Review of Predictors of Intrusive Memories of Distressing Events." *Psychological Bulletin* 144, no. 6 (2018): 584–640. doi.org/10.1037/bul0000132.

Nixon, Reginald D. V., Patricia A. Resick, and Michael G. Griffin. "Panic Following Trauma: The Etiology of Acute Posttraumatic Arousal." *Journal of Anxiety Disorders* 18, no. 2 (2004): 193–210. doi.org/10.1016/s0887-6185(02)00290-6.

Oulton, Jacinta M., Deryn Strange, Reginald D. V. Nixon, and Melanie K. T. Takarangi. "PTSD and the Role of Spontaneous Elaborative 'Nonmemories.'" *Psychology of Consciousness: Theory, Research, and Practice* 5, no. 4 (2018): 398–413. doi.org/10.1037/cns0000158.

Pietrzak, Robert H., Risë B. Goldstein, Steven M. Southwick, and Bridget F. Grant. "Prevalence and Axis I Comorbidity of Full and Partial Posttraumatic Stress Disorder in the United States: Results from Wave 2 of the National Epidemiologic Survey on Alcohol and Related Conditions." *Journal of Anxiety Disorders* 25, no. 3 (2011): 456–465. doi.org/10.1016/j.janxdis.2010.11.010.

Ramirez, Jennifer, Mollie Gordon, Mary Reissinger, Asim Shah, John Coverdale, and Phuong T. Nguyen. "The Importance of Maintaining Medical Professionalism While Experiencing Vicarious Trauma When Working with Human Trafficking Victims." *Traumatology*, 2020. doi.org/10.1037/trm0000248.

Sachser, Cedric, Ferdinand Keller, and Lutz Goldbeck. "Complex PTSD as Proposed for ICD-11: Validation of a New Disorder in Children and Adolescents and Their Response to Trauma-Focused Cognitive Behavioral Therapy." *Journal of Child Psychology and Psychiatry* 58, no. 2 (2016): 160–168. doi.org/10.1111/jcpp.12640.

Teng, Ellen J., Sara D. Bailey, Angelic D. Chaison, Nancy J. Petersen, Joseph D. Hamilton, and Nancy Jo Dunn. "Treating Comorbid Panic Disorder in Veterans with Posttraumatic Stress Disorder." *Journal of Consulting and Clinical Psychology* 76, no. 4 (2008): 704–710. doi.org/10.1037/0022-006x.76.4.710.

Weiss, Nicole H., Katherine L. Dixon-Gordon, Courtney Peasant, and Tami P. Sullivan. "An Examination of the Role of Difficulties Regulating Positive Emotions in Posttraumatic Stress Disorder." *Journal of Traumatic Stress* 31, no. 5 (2018): 775–780. doi.org/10.1002/jts.22330.

Chapter 4

Amstadter, Ananda B., and Laura L. Vernon. "Emotional Reactions During and After Trauma: A Comparison of Trauma Types." *Journal of Aggression, Maltreatment & Trauma* 16, no. 4 (2008): 391–408. doi.org/10.1080/10926770801926492.

Beck, Judith S. *Cognitive Behavior Therapy: Basics and Beyond*, 2nd edition. New York: Guilford Press, 2011.

Becker, C. B., & Zayfert, C. "Integrating DBT-Based Techniques and Concepts to Facilitate Exposure Treatment for PTSD." *Cognitive and Behavioral Practice* 8, no. 2 (2001): 107–122. doi.org/10.1016/s1077-7229(01)80017-1.

Difede, JoAnn, Megan Olden, and Judith Cukor. "Evidence-Based Treatment of Post-Traumatic Stress Disorder." *Annual Review of Medicine* 65 (2014): 319–332. doi.org/10.1146/annurev-med-051812-145438.

Dis, Eva A. M. van, Suzanne C. van Veen, Muriel A. Hagenaars, Neeltje M. Batelaan, Claudi L. H. Bockting, et al. "Long-Term Outcomes of Cognitive Behavioral Therapy for Anxiety-Related Disorders." *JAMA Psychiatry* 77, no. 3 (2020): 265–273. doi.org/10.1001/jamapsychiatry.2019.3986.

Ehring, Thomas, Renate Welboren, Nexhmedin Morina, Jelte M. Wicherts, Janina Freitag, and Paul M. G. Emmelkamp. "Meta-Analysis of Psychological Treatments for Posttraumatic Stress Disorder in Adult Survivors of Childhood Abuse." *Clinical Psychology Review* 34, no. 8 (2014): 645–657. doi.org/10.1016/j.cpr.2014.10.004.

Foa, Edna B., Jonathan D Huppert, and Shawn P. Cahill. "Emotional Processing Theory." In *Pathological Anxiety: Emotional Processing in Etiology and Treatment*, edited by Barbara Olasov Rothbaum, 4–34. New York: Guilford Press, 2006.

Heemstra, H. E. van, W. F. Scholte, T. Ehring, and P. A. Boelen. "Contextualizing Cognitions: The Relation Between Negative Post-Traumatic Cognitions and Post-Traumatic Stress Among Palestinian Refugees." *International Journal of Cognitive Therapy* 13, no. 2 (2020): 159–172. doi.org/10.1007/s41811-020-00066-7.

Hinton, Devon E., Stefan G. Hofmann, Edwin Rivera, Michael W. Otto, and Mark H. Pollack. "Culturally Adapted CBT (CA-CBT) for Latino Women with Treatment-Resistant PTSD: A Pilot Study Comparing CA-CBT to Applied Muscle Relaxation." *Behaviour Research and Therapy* 49, no. 4 (2011): 275–280. doi.org/10.1016/j.brat.2011.01.005.

Hofmann, Stefan G., Anu Asnaani, Imke J. J. Vonk, Alice T. Sawyer, and Angela Fang. "The Efficacy of Cognitive Behavioral Therapy: A Review of Meta-Analyses." *Cognitive Therapy and Research* 36, no. 5 (2012): 427–440. doi.org/10.1007/s10608-012-9476-1.

Ishikawa, Ryotaro. "Cognitive Behavioural Approaches for Post-Traumatic Stress Disorders." *Annals of Depression and Anxiety* 2, no. 3 (2015): 1–6.

Jensen, Tine K., Tonje Holt, Silje M. Ormhaug, Karina Egeland, Lene Granly, Live C. Hoaas, et al. "A Randomized Effectiveness Study Comparing Trauma-Focused Cognitive Behavioral Therapy with Therapy as Usual for Youth." *Journal of Clinical Child & Adolescent Psychology* 43, no. 3 (2013): 356–369. doi.org/10.1080/15374416.2013.822307.

Kar, Nilamadhab. "Cognitive Behavioral Therapy for the Treatment of Post-Traumatic Stress Disorder: A Review." *Neuropsychiatric Disease and Treatment* 2011, no. 7 (2011): 167–181. doi.org/10.2147/ndt.s10389.

Lancaster, Cynthia L., Jenni B. Teeters, Daniel F. Gros, and Sudie E. Back. "Posttraumatic Stress Disorder: Overview of Evidence-Based Assessment and Treatment." *Journal of Clinical Medicine* 5, no. 11 (2016). doi.org/10.3390/jcm5110105.

Resick, Patricia A., and Monica K. Schnicke. "Cognitive Processing Therapy for Sexual Assault Victims." *Journal of Consulting and Clinical Psychology* 60, no. 5 (1992): 748–756. doi.org/10.1037/0022-006x.60.5.748.

Scher, Christine D., Michael K. Suvak, and Patricia A. Resick. "Trauma Cognitions Are Related to Symptoms up to 10 Years after Cognitive Behavioral Treatment for Posttraumatic Stress Disorder." *Psychological Trauma: Theory, Research, Practice, and Policy* 9, no. 6 (2017): 750–757. doi.org/10.1037/tra0000258.

Shubina, Ivanna. "Cognitive-Behavioral Therapy of Patients with PTSD: Literature Review." *Procedia - Social and Behavioral Sciences* 165 (2015): 208–216. doi.org/10.1016/j.sbspro.2014.12.624.

Tuerk, Peter W., Bethany Wangelin, Sheila A. M. Rauch, Clara E. Dismuke, Matthew Yoder, Hugh Myrick, et al. "Health Service Utilization before and after Evidence-Based Treatment for PTSD." *Psychological Services* 10, no. 4 (2013): 401–409. doi.org/10.1037/a0030549.

Watkins, L. E., K. R. Sprang, and B. O. Rothbaum. "Treating PTSD: A Review of Evidence-Based Psychotherapy Interventions." *Frontiers in Behavioral Neuroscience* 12 (2018). doi.org/10.3389/fnbeh.2018.00258.

Zoellner, Lori A., Norah C. Feeny, Afsoon Eftekhari, and Edna B. Foa. "Changes in Negative Beliefs Following Three Brief Programs for Facilitating Recovery after Assault." *Depression and Anxiety* 28, no. 7 (2011): 532–540. doi.org/10.1002/da.20847.

Chapter 5

Blanaru, Monica, Boaz Bloch, Limor Vadas, Zahi Arnon, Naomi Ziv, Ilana Kremer, and Iris Haimov. "The Effects of Music Relaxation and Muscle Relaxation Techniques on Sleep Quality and Emotional Measures among Individuals with Posttraumatic Stress Disorder." *Mental Illness* 4, no. 2 (2012): 59–65. doi.org/10.4081/mi.2012.e13.

Dolbier, Christyn L., and Taylor E. Rush. "Efficacy of Abbreviated Progressive Muscle Relaxation in a High-Stress College Sample." *International Journal of Stress Management* 19, no. 1 (2012): 48–68. doi.org/10.1037/a0027326.

Dunsmoor, Joseph E., and Rony Paz. "Fear Generalization and Anxiety: Behavioral and Neural Mechanisms." *Biological Psychiatry* 78, no. 5 (2015): 336–343. doi.org/10.1016/j.biopsych.2015.04.010.

Hourani, Laurel, Stephen Tueller, Paul Kizakevich, Laura Strange, Gregory Lewis, Belinda Weimer, et al. "Effect of Stress Inoculation Training with Relaxation Breathing on Perceived Stress and Posttraumatic Stress Disorder in the Military: A Longitudinal Study." *International Journal of Stress Management* 25, no. S1 (2018): 124–136. doi.org/10.1037/str0000082.

Jacobs, Gregg D. "The Physiology of Mind–Body Interactions: The Stress Response and the Relaxation Response." *Journal of Alternative and Complementary Medicine* 7, no. S1 (2001): 83–92. doi.org/10.1089/107555301753393841.

Kantziari, Maria A., Nikolaos Nikolettos, Thomas Sivvas, Chryssa Tzoumaka Bakoula, George P. Chrousos, and Christina Darviri. "Stress Management during the Second Trimester of Pregnancy." *International Journal of Stress Management* 26, no. 1 (2019): 102–105. doi.org/10.1037/str0000078.

Kashani, Fahimeh, Sima Babaee, Masoud Bahrami, and Mahboobeh Valiani. "The Effects of Relaxation on Reducing Depression, Anxiety and Stress in Women Who Underwent Mastectomy for Breast Cancer." *Iranian Journal of Nursing and Midwifery Research* 17, no. 1 (2012): 30–33.

Manzoni, Gian Mauro, Francesco Pagnini, Gianluca Castelnuovo, and Enrico Molinari. "Relaxation Training for Anxiety: A Ten-Years Systematic Review with Meta-Analysis." *BMC Psychiatry* 8, no. 1 (2008). doi.org/10.1186/1471-244x-8-41.

Shirk, Stephen R., Patrice S. Crisostomo, Nathaniel Jungbluth, and Gretchen R. Gudmundsen. "Cognitive Mechanisms of Change in CBT for Adolescent Depression: Associations among Client Involvement, Cognitive Distortions, and Treatment Outcome." *International Journal of Cognitive Therapy* 6, no. 4 (2013): 311–324. doi.org/10.1521/ijct.2013.6.4.311.

Varvogli, Liza, and Christina Darviri. "Stress Management Techniques: Evidenced-Based Procedures that Reduce Stress and Promote Health." *Health Science Journal* 5, no. 2 (2011): 74–89.

Chapter 6

Beck, Judith S. *Cognitive Behavior Therapy: Basics and Beyond*, 2nd edition. New York: Guilford Press, 2011.

Dunsmoor, J. E., and R. Paz. "Fear Generalization and Anxiety: Behavioral and Neural Mechanisms." *Biological Psychiatry* 78, no. 5 (2015): 336–343. doi.org/10.1016/j.biopsych.2015.04.010.

Mueser, Kim T., Jennifer D. Gottlieb, Haiyi Xie, Weili Lu, Philip T. Yanos, Stanley D. Rosenberg, et al. "Evaluation of Cognitive Restructuring for Post-Traumatic Stress Disorder in People with Severe Mental Illness." *British Journal of Psychiatry* 206, no. 6 (2015): 501–508. doi.org/10.1192/bjp.bp.114.147926.

Mueser, Kim T., Stanley D. Rosenberg, and Harriet J. Rosenberg. "Trauma and Posttraumatic Stress Disorder in Vulnerable Populations." In *Treatment of Posttraumatic Stress Disorder in Special Populations: A Cognitive Restructuring Program*, 9–35. Washington, DC: American Psychological Association, 2009. doi.org/10.1037/11889-001.

Müller-Engelmann, Meike, and Regina Steil. "Cognitive Restructuring and Imagery Modification for Posttraumatic Stress Disorder (CRIM-PTSD): A Pilot Study." *Journal of Behavior Therapy and Experimental Psychiatry* 54 (2017): 44–50. doi.org/10.1016/j.jbtep.2016.06.004.

Najavits, Lisa M., Silke Gotthardt, Roger D. Weiss, and Marina Epstein. "Cognitive Distortions in the Dual Diagnosis of PTSD and Substance Use Disorder." *Cognitive Therapy and Research* 28, no. 2 (2004): 159–172. doi.org/10.1023/b:cotr.0000021537.18501.66.

O'Toole, Mia S., Douglas S. Mennin, Esben Hougaard, Robert Zachariae, and Nicole K. Rosenberg. "Cognitive and Emotion Regulation Change Processes in Cognitive Behavioural Therapy for Social Anxiety Disorder." *Clinical Psychology & Psychotherapy* 22, no. 6 (2014): 667–676. doi.org/10.1002/cpp.1926.

Panourgia, Constantina, and Amanda Comoretto. "Do Cognitive Distortions Explain the Longitudinal Relationship between Life Adversity and Emotional and Behavioural Problems in Secondary School Children?" *Stress & Health* 33, no. 5 (2017): 590–599. doi.org/10.1002/smi.2743.

Chapter 7

Baer, Ruth A. "Mindfulness, Assessment, and Transdiagnostic Processes." *Psychological Inquiry* 18, no. 4 (2007): 238–242. Accessed July 11, 2020. doi.org/10.1080/10478400701598306.

Bilican, F. Isil. "The Relationship between Focused Attention Meditation Practice Habits, Psychological Symptoms, and Quality of Life." *Journal of Religion & Health* 55, no. 6 (2016): 1980–1995. Accessed July 11, 2020. jstor.org/stable/44157057.

Boyd, Jenna E., Ruth A. Lanius, and Margaret C. McKinnon. "Mindfulness-Based Treatments for Posttraumatic Stress Disorder: A Review of the Treatment Literature and Neurobiological Evidence." *Journal of Psychiatry & Neuroscience* 43, no. 1 (2018): 7–25. doi.org/10.1503/jpn.170021.

Creswell, J. David, and Emily K. Lindsay. "How Does Mindfulness Training Affect Health? A Mindfulness Stress Buffering Account." *Current Directions in Psychological Science* 23, no. 6 (2014): 401–407. Accessed July 11, 2020. jstor.org/stable/44318808.

Gallegos, Autumn M., Megan C. Lytle, Jan A. Moynihan, and Nancy L. Talbot. "Mindfulness-Based Stress Reduction to Enhance Psychological Functioning and Improve Inflammatory Biomarkers in Trauma-Exposed Women: A Pilot Study." *Psychological Trauma: Theory, Research, Practice, and Policy* 7, no. 6 (2015): 525–532. doi.org/10.1037/tra0000053.

Hilton, L., A. R. Maher, B. Colaiaco, E. Apaydin, M. E. Sorbero, M. Booth, et al. "Meditation for Posttraumatic Stress: Systematic Review and Meta-Analysis." *Psychological Trauma: Theory, Research, Practice, and Policy* 9, no 4 (2017): 453–460. doi.org/10.1037/tra0000180.

Owens, Gina P., Kristen H. Walter, Kathleen M. Chard, and Paul A. Davis. "Changes in Mindfulness Skills and Treatment Response among Veterans in Residential PTSD Treatment." *Psychological Trauma: Theory, Research, Practice, and Policy* 4, no. 2 (2012): 221–228. doi.org/10.1037/a0024251.

Querstret, Dawn, Linda Morison, Sophie Dickinson, Mark Cropley, and Mary John. "Mindfulness-Based Stress Reduction and Mindfulness-Based Cognitive Therapy for Psychological Health and Well-Being in Nonclinical Samples: A Systematic Review and Meta-Analysis." *International Journal of Stress Management*, 2020. doi.org/10.1037/str0000165.

Shonin, Edo, William Van Gordon, and Mark D. Griffiths. "Does Mindfulness Work?" *British Medical Journal* 351 (2015). Accessed July 11, 2020. jstor.org/stable/26523903.

Smith, Bruce W., J. Alexis Ortiz, Laurie E. Steffen, Erin M. Tooley, Kathryn T. Wiggins, Elizabeth A. Yeater, et al. "Mindfulness Is Associated with Fewer PTSD Symptoms, Depressive Symptoms, Physical Symptoms, and Alcohol Problems in Urban Firefighters." *Journal of Consulting and Clinical Psychology* 79, no. 5 (2011): 613–617. doi.org/10.1037/a0025189.

Spijkerman, M. P. J., W. T. M. Pots, and E. T. Bohlmeijer. "Effectiveness of Online Mindfulness-Based Interventions in Improving Mental Health: A Review and Meta-Analysis of Randomised Controlled Trials." *Clinical Psychology Review* 45 (2016): 102–114. doi.org/10.1016/j.cpr.2016.03.009.

Vujanovic, A. A., B. Niles, A. Pietrefesa, S. K. Schmertz, and C. M. Potter. "Mindfulness in the Treatment of Posttraumatic Stress Disorder among Military Veterans." *Professional Psychology: Research and Practice* 42, no. 1 (2011): 24–31. doi.org/10.1037/a0022272.

Zelazo, Philip David, and Kristen E. Lyons. "Mindfulness Training in Childhood." *Human Development* 54, no. 2 (2011): 61–65. Accessed July 11, 2020. jstor.org/stable/26764991.

Chapter 8

Follette, Victoria M., Josef I. Ruzek, and Francis R. Abueg, eds. *Cognitive-Behavioral Therapies for Trauma*. New York: Guilford Press, 2006.

Jansen, Jens Einar, and Eric M. J. Morris. "Acceptance and Commitment Therapy for Posttraumatic Stress Disorder in Early Psychosis: A Case Series." *Cognitive and Behavioral Practice* 24, no. 2 (2017): 187–199. doi.org/10.1016/j.cbpra.2016.04.003.

Luoma, Jason B., and Melissa G. Platt. "Shame, Self-Criticism, Self-Stigma, and Compassion in Acceptance and Commitment Therapy." *Current Opinion in Psychology* 2 (2015): 97–101. doi.org/10.1016/j.copsyc.2014.12.016.

Chapter 9

Hendriks, Lotte, Rianne A. de Kleine, Theo G. Broekman, Gert-Jan Hendriks, and Agnes van Minnen. "Intensive Prolonged Exposure Therapy for Chronic PTSD Patients following Multiple Trauma and Multiple Treatment Attempts." *European Journal of Psychotraumatology* 9, no. 1 (2018): 1425574. doi.org/10.1080/20008198.2018.1425574.

Minnen, Agnes van, and Muriel Hagenaars. "Fear Activation and Habituation Patterns as Early Process Predictors of Response to Prolonged Exposure Treatment in PTSD." *Journal of Traumatic Stress* 15, no. 5 (2002): 359–367. doi.org/10.1023/a:1020177023209.

Norr, Aaron M., Kyle J. Bourassa, Elizabeth S. Stevens, Matthew J. Hawrilenko, Scott T. Michael, and Greg M. Reger. "Relationship between Change in In-Vivo Exposure Distress and PTSD Symptoms during Exposure Therapy for Active Duty Soldiers." *Journal of Psychiatric Research* 116 (2019): 133–137. doi.org/10.1016/j.jpsychires.2019.06.013.

Chapter 10

Alexander, Walter. "Pharmacotherapy for Post-Traumatic Stress Disorder in Combat Veterans." *Pharmacy and Therapeutics* 37, no. 1 (2012): 32–38.

Friedman, Matthew J., and Nancy C. Bernardy. "Considering Future Pharmacotherapy for PTSD." *Neuroscience Letters* 649 (2016): 181–185. doi.org/10.1016/j.neulet .2016.11.048.

Jeffreys, Matt. "Clinician's Guide to Medications for PTSD." July 1, 2009. Washington, DC: US Department of Veterans Affairs. ptsd.va.gov/professional/treat/txessentials /clinician_guide_meds.asp.

Kozarić-Kovačić, Dragica. "Psychopharmacotherapy of Posttraumatic Stress Disorder." *Croatian Medical Journal* 49, no. 4 (2008): 459–475. doi.org/10.3325/cmj.2008.4.459.

Martenyi, Ferenc, Eileen B. Brown, Harry Zhang, Stephanie C. Koke, and Apurva Prakash. "Fluoxetine v. Placebo in Prevention of Relapse in Post-Traumatic Stress Disorder." *British Journal of Psychiatry* 181, no. 4 (2002): 315–320. doi.org/10.1192/bjp.181.4.315.

Nappi, Carla M., Sean P. A. Drummond, and Joshua M. H. Hall. "Treating Nightmares and Insomnia in Posttraumatic Stress Disorder: A Review of Current Evidence." *Neuropharmacology* 62, no. 2 (2012): 576–585. doi.org/10.1016/j.neuropharm.2011.02.029.

Schneier, Franklin R., Yuval Neria, Martina Pavlicova, Elizabeth Hembree, Eun Jung Suh, Lawrence Amsel, and Randall D. Marshall. "Combined Prolonged Exposure Therapy and Paroxetine for PTSD Related to the World Trade Center Attack: A Randomized Controlled Trial." *American Journal of Psychiatry* 169, no. 1 (2012): 80–88. doi.org/10.1176 /appi.ajp.2011.11020321.

Stein, Dan J., Ron Pedersen, Barbara O. Rothbaum, David S. Baldwin, Saeeduddin Ahmed, Jeff Musgnung, and Jonathan Davidson. "Onset of Activity and Time to Response on Individual CAPS-SX$_{17}$ Items in Patients Treated for Post-Traumatic Stress Disorder with Venlafaxine ER: A Pooled Analysis." *International Journal of Neuropsychopharmacology* 12, no. 1 (2009): 23–31. doi.org/10.1017/s1461145708008961.

Zhang, Ye, Rong Ren, Larry D. Sanford, Linghui Yang, Yuenan Ni, Junying Zhou, et al. "The Effects of Prazosin on Sleep Disturbances in Post-Traumatic Stress Disorder: A Systematic Review and Meta-Analysis." *Sleep Medicine* 67 (2020): 225–231. doi.org/10.1016 /j.sleep.2019.06.010.

Zoellner, Lori A., Peter P. Roy-Byrne, Matig Mavissakalian, and Norah C. Feeny. "Doubly Randomized Preference Trial of Prolonged Exposure Versus Sertraline for Treatment of PTSD." *American Journal of Psychiatry* 176, no. 4 (2019): 287–296. doi.org/10.1176 /appi.ajp.2018.17090995.

Chapter 12

Bensimon, Moshe. "Elaboration on the Association between Trauma, PTSD and Posttraumatic Growth: The Role of Trait Resilience." *Personality and Individual Differences* 52, no. 7 (2012): 782–787. doi.org/10.1016/j.paid.2012.01.011.

Cobb, Amanda R., Richard G. Tedeschi, Lawrence G. Calhoun, and Arnie Cann. "Correlates of Posttraumatic Growth in Survivors of Intimate Partner Violence." *Journal of Traumatic Stress* 19, no. 6 (2006): 895–903. doi.org/10.1002/jts.20171.

Harbin, Ami. "Prescribing Posttraumatic Growth." *Bioethics* 29, no. 9 (2015): 671–679. doi.org/10.1111/bioe.12164.

Joseph, Stephen, David Murphy, and Stephen Regel. "An Affective-Cognitive Processing Model of Post-Traumatic Growth." *Clinical Psychology & Psychotherapy* 19, no. 4 (2012): 316–325. doi.org/10.1002/cpp.1798.

Kobasa, Suzanne, S. R. Maddi, and S. Kahn. "Hardiness and Health: A Prospective Study." *Journal of Personality and Social Psychology* 42, no. 1 (1982): 168–177. doi.org/10.1037/0022-3514.42.1.168.

Sheridan, Grace, and Alan Carr. "Survivors' Lived Experiences of Posttraumatic Growth after Institutional Childhood Abuse: An Interpretative Phenomenological Analysis." *Child Abuse & Neglect* 103 (2020): 104430. doi.org/10.1016/j.chiabu.2020.104430.

Ssenyonga, Joseph, Vicki Owens, and David Kani Olema. "Posttraumatic Growth, Resilience, and Posttraumatic Stress Disorder (PTSD) among Refugees." *Procedia - Social and Behavioral Sciences* 82 (2013): 144–148. doi.org/10.1016/j.sbspro.2013.06.238.

Tedeschi, Richard G., and Lawrence G. Calhoun. "Posttraumatic Growth: Conceptual Foundations and Empirical Evidence." *Psychological Inquiry* 15, no. 1 (2004): 1–18. Accessed July 11, 2020. jstor.org/stable/20447194.

Index